MANAGE YOUR MENOPAUSE
2 BOOKS IN 1

HOW TO BALANCE HORMONES
AND PREVENT MIDDLE-AGE SPREAD

By Silvana Siskov

Thank you for purchasing
Manage Your Menopause
2 Books in 1

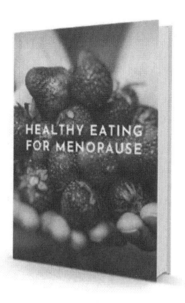

Please visit <u>bit.ly/menopause-healthy-recipes-2</u>
and download
Healthy Eating for Menopause – Recipe Book.
You will find plenty of delicious recipes there to
help you achieve a confident body.

MANAGE YOUR MENOPAUSE 2 BOOKS IN 1
BEAT YOUR MENOPAUSE WEIGHT GAIN
FREE YOURSELF FROM HOT FLUSHES AND NIGHT SWEATS
www.silvanasiskov.com

Table of Contents

BEAT YOUR MENOPAUSE WEIGHT GAIN

Balance Hormones, Stop Middle-Age Spread, Boost Your Health and Vitality

By Silvana Siskov

Introduction

Let's be honest; it is fabulous to be a woman, but it is not easy.

You are busy having fun when you are young and then suddenly your period comes along, shocking you to the core. Then, you just about get the hang of periods when they suddenly stop, signalling that there is a new life growing inside of you. Perhaps you are pregnant once, twice or maybe not at all, but then as you start to settle down, everything changes again and you begin to notice hot flushes, night sweats, weight gain, mood swings. Then, your period stops abruptly.

Yes, life as a woman is full of ups and downs and we have those pesky hormones to thank for it.

The fact you have picked up this book tells me that you are somewhere over the age of 40 and you are possibly wondering what is happening to your body. Do not worry, this happens to all of us and while reaching the age of menopause is not exactly a barrel of laughs, it is a natural part of every woman's life cycle.

The aim of this book is to help you through one of the most troublesome symptoms related to the menopause — weight gain. I know first-hand how difficult this phase of life can be. Not only are you experiencing changes within your body, but you are coming to terms with the fact that you are getting older and are no longer able to become pregnant. Though this is a natural part of the ageing process, it is a lot to take in and can be extremely traumatic for some women to handle.

The changes that the menopause can bring can easily affect the way you see yourself, the way you feel and your self-confidence, but it does not have to be such a negative experience. There are plenty of hints and tricks you can use to overcome some of the symptoms and effects this natural phase of life can bring.

Weight gain can be one of the most common and distressing parts of the menopause. By learning how to approach it positively, you can overcome the possible weight increase and successfully manage the other effects brought on by the menopause.

During this phase of your life, visceral fat is most common, leading to fat accumulations around the abdomen and collections around the internal organs. This increases your risk of developing serious health issues, such as type 2 diabetes, if left unchecked. Therefore, taking action is crucial. Apart from causing problems with your health, this also damages your confidence, because any type of weight gain can cause you to feel less than your best, sluggish and down.

Most women notice that as they enter the menopause, they start to gain weight more easily than before, and when they try to lose it, the entire process is much harder than it was in their earlier years. Not knowing the right ways to shift this fat can lead you to feel worse about yourself, which is not an enjoyable experience when combined with the other effects of the menopause.

Life is too short to spend time worrying and being upset about the menopause; you simply need to take advice and find ways to avoid or overcome the worst effects. That is where I can help.

I want to show you that while the menopause is inevitable, it does not need to be an end to your years of feeling beautiful, attractive and full of life. Those years can continue and become even better — once everything settles down. Remember, you are still the same strong and independent woman you were before the menopause arrived; it is just that a few bodily changes are happening that are causing you to feel a little less like yourself at present. However, this feeling will begin to change, and you will start to feel like yourself again.

The menopause can be a time for you to realise your power and use it as a springboard towards getting what you really want out of life. By focusing on health and well-being, you can feel better in yourself and open new doors of opportunity. Who knows what changes will come your way as a result of all this brimming confidence? You are giving yourself a chance to start over and do the things you never did before; it is a second chance to live your life to the full.

You do not have to deny yourself the things you enjoy to lose the menopause-related weight. You do not have to avoid looking in the mirror, and you do not have to think about your age and allow it to turn your mindset towards the negative end of the scale. Instead, why not let me show you the way forward? It is a decision you will not regret.

You will learn not only how to avoid menopausal weight gain and lose any weight you might have noticed creeping on, but also how to view the menopause as something that is just happening *to you*, not as something which is there to define you as a woman.

I know how you feel. I have been there myself and have helped countless women just like you to cope with this challenging yet surmountable time of life. All you need to do is keep an open mind, focus on the positive aspects of the menopause experience and read on.

Chapter 1

Perimenopause, Menopause, and Postmenopause — What Is It All About?

By reading and following the advice I give you in this book, not only will you learn to view the menopause through positive eyes, but you will also learn what you need to do to avoid the weight gain that so many women face around this period of life.

I will not lie and tell you that the menopause will be a breeze for all women. We are all unique in our own and extraordinary ways and that means there is never going to be a one size fits all answer to any health approach. Women have been going through what we affectionately call "the change" for centuries, so we are well placed to understand what is going on and learn from their experience and successfully overcome some of the challenging effects.

Perimenopause, Menopause, and Postmenopause — What do These Terms Mean?

Before we delve into the finer details of the menopause, I must first arm you with the knowledge and understanding required. You need to understand what the terms I am going to use mean, i.e. perimenopause, menopause and postmenopause. Only then can you properly understand not only what I am talking about, but what it means for you.

This chapter is focusing on giving you basic but very important information about the three menopausal phases.

Before we delve into the main issue here, i.e. how to avoid menopausal weight gain, you need to have some background knowledge. You might already know something about the menopause through talking to other women or doing your own research, but for the sake of clarity, let's go through some of the basics.

Remember that information on the internet about anything health-related can be unreliable; anyone can publish information online, and it does not have to be fact-checked. However, you know that you can trust the information in this book and will not need to carry out any Google searches for clarification.

What Is the Difference Between the Perimenopause and the Menopause?

The perimenopause is the time before the actual menopause is established. During this time, you may experience a range of different symptoms. It is not unusual for periods to stop and start, or feel perfectly "normal" one day and be overwhelmed with the menopausal symptoms that can make you feel miserable or anxious the following day. Many women have mistakenly thought they were pregnant, only to find out later that they were perimenopausal, and vice versa.

In the following chapter, I am going to talk in more detail about the symptoms of the perimenopause and the menopause, as it is crucial to understand that during this period of a woman's life, hormonal imbalance can cause so many issues and can turn your life upside down. You will learn more about this as you read through this book.

The perimenopausal period, loosely translated as "around the menopause" can last for a few years. In some cases, it may last anything up to 10 years. This stage runs into the actual menopause itself when your periods stop entirely.

The first sign that you are perimenopausal and therefore heading towards the menopause comes in the shape of irregular periods. Your regular pattern may show changes, e.g. your periods might be lighter or heavier than before. You might start to have them more frequently or they can become less frequent and have no actual pattern. This can be extremely bothersome, as you have no way to predict when your period is due. Going away on holiday can be troublesome because you cannot plan when Mother Nature is going to come calling.

The perimenopause usually starts in a woman's forties, but in some cases it can begin earlier, in the late thirties. It is possible, though unusual, for some women to start in their twenties. There is no way of knowing when your particular menopausal period will start. There is some suggestion that you should look to your mother and when she began to go through her "change", but again, we are all unique, and that means there is no menopausal crystal ball for us to predict the start of the menopause. In my family, my mother had her last period around her 55th birthday. My sister is 55 now, and she is following in my mother's steps. But my situation is very different — I had my last period at the age of 49. So, do we all need to look at our mothers to know when we will begin with the "change"? No. We can never know exactly when it will happen.

So, if the perimenopause is the time before the menopause, what is the actual menopause?

Menopause is easy to define — this is the point when your ovaries stop releasing eggs. At this stage, your periods will stop completely. You will no longer be able to get pregnant naturally, and your reproductive years are now behind you.

A Word about Postmenopause

Once the menopause is over, i.e. once you have not had a period for one full year (assuming you are 50 or over, and two full years if you are under 50), you enter the postmenopausal phase. As the name suggests, this is the time after you experienced the menopause, but that does not necessarily mean that all your symptoms will magically disappear.

It is not unusual for some women to continue to experience symptoms for up to 10 years afterwards. However, during this time the symptoms are usually a little less severe. They will begin to diminish gradually as time goes on, leaving you free to enjoy life without hot flushes and other annoying issues that the menopause can bring your way.

These uncomfortable symptoms occur because the former levels of oestrogen and progesterone have dropped, which is what caused the menopause in the first place.

The good news is that you will not have menstruation anymore, and the presence of periods in your life is now completely behind you. You will be able to enjoy greater freedom in all your activities such as going swimming at any time of the month. If you do notice any bleeding and you are definitely in the postmenopausal phase, you should see your doctor for a checkup.

You are Currently Being Controlled by Your Hormones

Hormones are extremely powerful, but we tend to underrate their influence on our body's functions. They help to regulate our weight (more on that shortly), mood, sleep, growth and a broad range of other tasks that add to our overall health and well-being. We need to look in more detail at the two main hormones controlling menopause; they are called oestrogen and progesterone. Decreased levels of these two hormones during the menopause can cause many unpleasant symptoms.

These hormones are also connected to your menstrual cycle. However, as we become a little older, our levels of these hormones begin to drop. When this happens, our hormonal balance is totally out of sync, which is why you may experience a variety of symptoms during this time, such as mood swings or agitation.

Depending upon the severity of your symptoms, your doctor may suggest that you start Hormone Replacement Therapy (HRT) to help you balance your hormones. HRT effectively replaces the hormones that are low due to the approaching menopause. However, that is a choice that every woman must decide for herself and you should read about the pros and cons of this treatment before you make a final decision.

This book is not about treatment for the menopause. Therefore, I am not going to dwell on HRT. However, for the sake of clarity it has to be mentioned.

If you want to learn more about different menopausal symptoms and how to handle them, my book, *Free Yourself From Hot Flushes and Night Sweats: The Essential Guide to a Happy And Healthy Menopause* might be an interesting read for you. In this book you will discover how to reduce your hot flushes and night sweats and find out about the effects of the menopause on your libido. You will learn many ways to deal with the menopause and its associated symptoms by making smart lifestyle changes, so you can approach the menopause with the right mindset.

If you are managing the effects of the menopause well and simply want to avoid weight gain, which is often one of the main factors affecting a woman's confidence and causing damage to her health, then the rest of this book will undoubtedly be of interest to you.

What you need to understand at this point is that hormones, or a lack thereof, control every aspect of your menopausal experience. This is a natural part of the ageing process for a woman and while it can be difficult to understand or deal with, take heart in the fact that it is normal.

It is easy to become scared or worried about what is happening to your body when you are starting to notice changes, but remember that you are simply going through a natural process. Recognising this should help you deal with any anxiety you experience and leave you free to focus on one burning topic....

Why Does All of This Lead to Weight Gain?

Ah, the very crux of this book!

Unfortunately, the hormonal ups and downs happening during the perimenopausal and menopausal stages mean that you will probably notice a little weight gain. During this time, most women see that they are putting weight on without even trying.

You are probably not eating anything different and you feel that you are not moving any less, but the scales begin to creep up a little. You will probably notice this particularly around your midriff; this is the visceral fat that I talked about in the introductory section.

There are two things to pay attention to here — firstly, the confidence issue. There are not many women who are happy to put on weight and simply live with it. It is bound to dent your confidence a little, especially if you are noticing extra pounds without having done anything to deserve it! Let's be honest, if you have been away on holiday and enjoyed the cakes and wine a little too much, you know that you are going to have to cut back when you get home, but if you have done nothing, to cause this change; it is quite a shock!

Weight gain can have an extremely damaging effect on the way you feel about yourself in general. Some women may have had a weight problem in the past, battled to lose it and felt proud of their efforts (rightly so), only to find that their hormones want to undo their hard work when the menopausal period begins. Quite understandably, this can be upsetting and extremely discouraging, affecting not only your confidence but also harming your self-worth.

The second important aspect is that visceral fat can be injurious to your health because it accumulates around the internal organs. This may increase the possibility of you developing chronic diseases and severe health conditions such as heart disease, diabetes, stroke, high blood pressure, high cholesterol levels and liver problems. These are just a few examples of serious health issues, which can damage your quality of life and may even prove to be fatal. We need to do everything we can to reduce these risk factors, to ensure that we all live long and healthy lives.

The problem is that this menopausal weight gain can be harder to shift than the weight gain from your younger age. For some reason, you put weight on more easily, yet it will not go away without a fight! It is surely one of life's rather unpleasant ironies.

By understanding why this is happening you can work out ways to overcome this problem, and I promise you, it can be beaten!

To understand it, let's delve a little deeper.

Many studies show that during the menopause the two main female sex hormones — oestrogen and progesterone, start fluctuating. These hormone changes can lead to developing excess weight around the middle.

During this time of your life, your testosterone levels will also decrease, leading to muscle mass loss. Testosterone is the male sex hormone but women have it too. When you lose muscle, your body will no longer be able to burn fat fast and you will gain weight easily. This happens naturally as you grow older and unless you are in the gym every day pumping iron (nobody has time for that), it is something you are certainly going to notice.

Hormonal imbalance during the menopause is known to cause increased appetite and higher calorie intake. Many women have higher fasting insulin levels and insulin resistance during this period of their lives. This can significantly affect the rate of their metabolism. It causes their metabolism to slow down, and this affects how fast they burn fat. The fact is, the slower you burn fat, the more fat you have; the quicker you burn fat, the less fat you have. A slower metabolism has an adverse effect on the function of the postmenopausal body.

In addition to regulating the menstrual cycle, oestrogen is a hormone which is also responsible for managing your weight and ensuring that your metabolism is functioning correctly. It impacts the amount of fat in the body.

As you move through the perimenopause and into the menopause, the slow decline of oestrogen (a type called estradiol in particular) can cause your body to store more fat. This results in weight gain and has a potentially harmful effect on bone density, leading to osteoporosis and poor heart health.

Hormonal imbalances caused by the menopause can affect your sleep quality, and if you are sleep deprived, you are more likely to make poor food choices and reduce the amount of exercise you are doing, simply because you are so tired. Lack of sleep will also affect your "hunger" hormones known as leptin and ghrelin. These two hormones are known to influence your hunger level and increase your appetite.

As you will learn later on in this book, sleep disruption is one of the menopause symptoms, so, yet again we have another trigger for the weight-increase to deal with.

However, do not despair, because I have plenty of advice on handling this problem and keeping your weight in check. What you need to do is to focus your time and attention on becoming healthier, eliminating unhealthy habits, and making good, firm, and positive choices instead.

Eating healthy and moving your body more are the two main good habits that can help control your menopausal weight gain, in addition to several other factors. In this book, we will explore some of those factors and look at what you need to do to achieve your weight loss goal.

Learning to See the Menopause From a Positive Perspective

If there is one thing I understand more than anything else on this subject, it is just how detrimental the menopause can be to some women's emotional health. It is a rollercoaster that you think will never end and while at the back of your mind you know that it will, in reality, it seems as though it will always be in your life, controlling your every move and every thought.

It has been quite a few years since I went through the "change", when I felt totally drained and overwhelmed by my menopausal symptoms, but I still remember thinking "I can't go through life feeling like this anymore". Since then, I have learnt a lot about the menopause and how to handle its symptoms. I wish I had known then what I know now. At the time I felt like it was never going to end, but remember this — you have control, you just need to take it back!

Putting on weight and noticing changes in your body, as well as the realisation that your reproductive years are coming to an end, can impact a woman's confidence levels. Lack of confidence can easily lead you down negative roads, such as turning to food or drinking too much to deal with the way this deficit makes you feel.

Emotional eating is often a choice that many women make to help them cope with their problems. The difficulty with seeking comfort in overeating is that it does not solve any problems. This impulsive behaviour usually makes the situation much worse than before.

Self-care is crucial during this time of your life. There are many healthy outlets for your emotions. It is vital that you look towards these, rather than overeating, smoking, or drinking too much. These coping devices will simply cause your weight to increase even more, further compounding your lack of confidence and making the entire problem much worse. When you think negatively, you feel negative; when you think positively and make positive life choices, you feel more positive and therefore much happier. This has a knock-on effect on every aspect of your life, your health included.

I suggest you speak to a friend, look for support networks in your local community, take your mind off what is going on within your body and instead look towards positivity. Yes, your body is changing, and yes, this does mean that you are no longer fertile, but hopefully, by this age, you were not thinking about having more children anyway. The thought of this is likely to make you shudder, but even if it does not, consider this your freedom card.

No more periods, no more PMS, the freedom to go swimming and stay in the water as long as you like and wear white as much as you like. These might seem like small things, but when you have spent a lifetime so far dealing with them, the freedom might be quite refreshing!

The menopause does not have to define you and it does not have to be a full stop to anything. It is merely something that is happening within your body, and with time you will simply go about your life as before, or perhaps with even more confidence as you realise your true capabilities.

Key Points

This has been an informational chapter to help you understand more about the perimenopausal phase and why it is different from the actual menopause. You were also introduced to the term "postmenopause".

You cannot learn how to handle and deal with something unless you realise what is going on and why. Hopefully, by this point, you have gained a clearer picture of what this time in your life is about, and you have realised that this is a normal process in every woman's life.

The aim of this book is to teach you how to avoid and reduce weight gain during the menopause and to educate you about the role of hormones and their influence on your weight.

The main points to remember from this chapter are:

- The perimenopause is the period before the actual menopause.

- Most women enter the perimenopause in their forties. However, this can be as early as their late thirties or even sooner in some cases.

- Every woman is unique.

- The menopause occurs when your ovaries no longer release eggs and you are therefore no longer fertile.

- The two critical female hormones are oestrogen and progesterone, and during this time, they begin to fall gradually.

- Hormones have a crucial role in regulating many different bodily functions, including sleep and metabolism.

- As oestrogen levels fall, your metabolism slows down. This can lead to weight gain as well as potentially affecting your sleep levels. Sleep deprivation can affect your "hunger" hormones and cause you to gain weight due to poor food choices.

- Weight gain during the menopause can be managed and overcome provided you make changes to your diet and lifestyle.

Chapter 2

Signs the Menopause is Around the Corner

Now that you know what the perimenopause and menopause are, we need to talk about the symptoms. This will help you to identify when this time of life is coming your way, or whether you might already be there.

Remember, every woman is different, which means you may experience all of the symptoms I am going to talk about, or you may only experience a few. You might be fortunate and barely experience any at all. The average woman could experience several common symptoms for up to a decade before the ovaries stop releasing eggs and the whole process is complete.

You might be slightly perturbed by the list of symptoms I am about to talk about, but remember that these can be mild, moderate, and rarely severe. If you are experiencing severe symptoms that affect your quality of life, consult your doctor and find out if any treatment options might help you cope a little better.

The other piece of good news is that this list of symptoms is unlikely to be constant. You might experience them on some days, most days for a month, and then none for a while. There is no way to predict how the menopause is going to impact you in terms of symptoms and severity, but it is vital to know what is normal and what is not.

Signs of the Perimenopausal Period

The most common signs that you are heading towards menopause, i.e. you are in the perimenopausal stage are the following:

- **Experiencing hot flushes** – Hot flushes are sudden and very short sensations of heat, which creep up your chest, into your neck and up to your face. You might also look flushed, i.e. a little red in the face, and you might even sweat. However, you might simply feel like you are red and sweaty but show no external signs at all. Some women suffer severely with hot flushes. They might get soaking wet within 10 seconds, but then they could spend the next 60 seconds freezing due to the changes in their body temperature.

- *Night sweats* – Alongside the hot flushes that usually occur while awake, you may also experience night sweats. These tend to wake you up unexpectedly and mimic the sensation of a hot flush. They disappear as quickly as they come, but by that point you are already awake, boiling hot, soaking wet and your night's sleep is disturbed. As soon as the night sweat disappears, you are freezing cold and searching for the extra blanket.

- *Sleep problems* – Aside from the night sweats, you may notice that you have difficulty nodding off to sleep at night, or you wake up frequently. This is due to the falling hormone levels, especially oestrogen, which affect your relaxation and sleep routine. As a result, you are likely to be irritable the next day and lack energy because you have missed out on a good night's sleep. You will most probably turn to sugary foods in order to regain your strength. The longer this cycle continues, the worse the next day symptoms become.

- **Vaginal dryness and discomfort** – This is caused by the falling hormone levels, which can cause vaginal dryness and discomfort during sex. This may sometimes lead to itching and soreness in the vaginal area, and some women notice that they also experience more yeast infections during this time. If you notice these symptoms, try using a lubricant during sex to make the experience more comfortable and to avoid soreness.

- **More urinary tract infections (UTIs)** – Some women are more prone to UTIs than others. If you notice you are experiencing more of these rather irritating occurrences during the perimenopausal period than before, a consultation with your doctor is necessary.

- **Issues with concentration and forgetfulness** – Many women notice that they suddenly develop a case of "baby brain" – without the baby – during this time. We can blame hormones once more here, but it could also be due to the lack of sleep.

- **Experiencing palpitations** – Falling oestrogen levels or fluctuations during the perimenopause can often lead to palpitations. During palpitations your heart will be pounding and beating fast for a few seconds. You must remain calm if you experience these. Practising yoga and meditation are known to be great for making you feel more relaxed which can help with palpitations. I advise you to visit your doctor if you experience this problem regularly. Keep in mind that changes in hormone levels are typically connected to increased palpitations.

- **Headaches** – Headaches are another side effect of your hormones being totally out of sync at this time. However, if you have severe headaches or migraines, do consult your doctor; it might have nothing to do with the menopause!

- **Weight gain** – The very subject of this book. Reduced muscle mass resulting in weight gain is one of the most common complaints from menopausal women, and we already know that visceral fat can be dangerous. Many women also notice a change in their general body shape at this time. By focusing on lifestyle changes, which I will discuss as we move through the coming chapters, you will be more in control of managing your weight during the menopause.

Remember, just because you are not experiencing *all* of the symptoms above, it does not mean there is anything wrong; every woman is different.

When Is the Menopause Over?

How will you know when you finished with the menopause and the postmenopause started?

Good question!

It is easy to say you have completed the menopause once you feel yourself again and are no longer experiencing symptoms, but those pesky hormones might not have got the memo. There may be fluctuations in your hormone levels after the menopause is over. If that does happen, the symptoms are likely to be mild and possibly unnoticeable.

I have already mentioned and it is worth mentioning again — you are considered postmenopausal after your periods have stopped entirely for two years if you are under the age of 50 and for one year if you are over the age of 50. That means no periods for one or two years straight, depending upon your age. By that time, you will also notice that most of the symptoms have reduced or disappeared. A few women experience severe symptoms for some years, but this is unusual, and most return to their normal self shortly after entering the postmenopause.

The postmenopause may bring its own challenges; there is no phase in a woman's life free of challenges, but the perimenopausal stage seems to affect women's well-being the most. A variety of unpleasant symptoms that we face during this period is something that many women struggle with. Some women argue that the menopause is the most difficult time of their lives due to experiencing physical symptoms and going through psychological and emotional changes, which affect their health, confidence and general well-being.

Let's explore this further in the next section.

How the Menopause May Affect Your Confidence?

The menopause is not just about the physical symptoms you are experiencing; it is also about how it makes you feel about yourself. Never underestimate just how important your confidence is in life — it affects a whole range of areas: your motivation to make changes to your relationships, self-worth and a host of other unexpected things. Self-confidence in life is key, and it can be affected by the smallest thing.

Whenever we go through significant life changes, it is easy to be knocked off-kilter and experience a minor confidence crisis. Some women sail through the menopause, but more tend to struggle a little with confidence at some stage. You are not alone if you are struggling with the menopause. Never feel that you simply have to woman up and deal with it; this is a big issue in your life and you need to progress through it in a way that feels right to you and to find support from those around you.

It is normal to be affected by this massive change in life, but that does not mean that you should dwell on the negatives. Every woman has a different symptom that causes them the most trouble. For some, it could be the lack of energy and tiredness, due to those fluctuating hormones. For others, it could be weight gain, or it could be feeling agitated. The entire cocktail of hormonal effects leaves you open to potential mood changes, and it can also drastically affect the way you think of yourself inside. This is likely to cause you to feel a different sense of self. Your confidence will take a hit as a result, because you may have developed a different perspective.

Many women start to worry that they are no longer attractive, but the truth is that a menopausal woman is no less and no more beautiful than a woman who is yet to go through the menopause. Whether or not you are able to menstruate has no bearing on your beauty both inside or out! Look at some of the sexiest stars in the celebrity world, perhaps Jennifer Lopez, as one example — she is over 50, and she is undoubtedly still attractive and sexy! Attractiveness and sexiness have nothing to do with your ability to carry a child, your ability to menstruate and certainly nothing to with your ability to release an egg from your ovaries every month!

You are just as beautiful as you were before you started the menopause, and that is not going to change because of your hormones. Once the menopause is over, many women reclaim their confidence to the point where they never look back. There is nothing sexier or more attractive than a woman who is comfortable in her body, owning her sexuality and someone who exudes confidence in who she is. That is a cocktail for real confidence and happiness right there! It does not matter how old or young she is, or whether she is menopausal or not. What matters is the way she feels about herself.

However, I want you to know that if you do feel a little lacking in confidence at this stage of your life, it is entirely normal. Many women feel this way, and there is nothing wrong with you if you are not feeling your very best. Life changes can knock us sideways sometimes, and hormones are powerful things. It is not easy to battle hormones every single day and get up and go about your business at the same time. You should pat yourself on the back for having the power to do just that. All you need to do is carry on doing what you are doing for a little longer, with perhaps a few changes to your outlook and lifestyle to battle any weight gain issues.

Of course, emotions are just as powerful as hormones. If you are genuinely struggling, seek help from your loved ones, look for support networks of women who are also going through the same time in life as you, or have a chat with your doctor if you are feeling low. There is help out there, and even though feeling down and lacking in confidence at this stage of life is quite common, you do not have to live with it.

Before I end this chapter, it is important to mention that the lifestyle changes I will discuss throughout the rest of the book will go a long way to giving you back your power and, therefore, your confidence. When you take ownership of your health and your body, you step into your power. This fuels your confidence and helps you to understand just how strong you really are.

Key Points

There is a range of symptoms that signal you are in the menopausal period of your life, but it is vital to remember that every woman is different, so you might not experience all of them or even many of them. Symptoms can vary in severity too, so if you are particularly struggling with one symptom, seek help from your doctor to find ways to reduce its effect on your life.

Women find the main issue with the menopause is often not the symptoms, but the effects that it can have on their confidence. The idea of going through the menopause can easily cause a woman to feel bad about herself, and when you add to the mix weight gain and sleep deprivation, the whole thing can become a rather unpleasant experience. The good news is that throughout this book, I am going to give you actionable, easy to follow advice on how to reduce the effects, thereby helping you to look and feel your best throughout the menopause and beyond.

The main points to remember from this chapter are:

- You have completed the menopause when you have had no periods for two years straight if you are under the age of 50, or one year if you are over this age.

- Menopausal symptoms can range in severity, from mild to severe.

- Every woman will experience a different combination of symptoms.

- If you struggle with symptoms, it is important to seek help to reduce their effects.

- The menopause itself can easily affect a woman's confidence, especially if she gains weight.

- Fluctuations in hormones can cause havoc with how you feel, so it is vital to take it easy on yourself.

- You are just as beautiful *now* as you were *before* the menopause — the menopause does not dictate your beauty or your worth.

Chapter 3

Stress, Weight Gain and the Menopause

How many times per day do you utter the words "I am so stressed?" and how many times do you hear other people around you saying it?

Probably a lot.

We tend to say we are stressed most of the time when the reality is that we are not. We do not take stress as seriously as we should. Did you know that stress can be life-threatening when left to grow over the long term? It sounds dramatic, but it is true. You will come to realise how, as I talk more about why it is dangerous and what detrimental impact stress can have. However, a little pressure can be useful because it serves as a motivator.

Confused?

Do not be.

A little stress is useful in some cases, but when stress is allowed to build up and last over a long period, it can be extremely damaging. It can damage your mental and physical state.

How does this link to the menopause?

Menopause can be a stressful time for a woman. If you are struggling with menopausal symptoms, unhappy with weight gain, and generally feeling low in confidence and mood, the stress will easily creep into your life and cause everything to seem so much more strenuous and hard to cope with.

Everyone has been through a period of real stress at some point in their lives. Can you remember how it felt for you? You probably could not concentrate for very long and you might have had trouble sleeping. Maybe you even turned to overeating or adopted another damaging way to handle the emotions you were experiencing? You probably snapped at everyone in your close vicinity and might have ended up having arguments for no reason whatsoever.

It is common to feel more stress at this time of your life, simply because you might be lacking in sleep, you feel confused or worried about what is going on inside your body (or in your life in general), your hormones are all over the place, and everything seems a little out of control. You may be experiencing brain fog too, and your memory does not seem to be as sharp as it used to be. While going through the menopause can itself cause weight gain, surprisingly so can stress. That means that managing a healthy weight could be even more difficult than when you are younger.

It is common for menopausal women to face many stressful events in addition to the changes they experience inside their bodies. Stressful events that are most prevalent for women in their forties and fifties are associated with children leaving home, going through a divorce, or taking care of elderly parents. Any of these events can bring a tremendous amount of stress.

In this chapter, I am going to talk to you about what stress is and the stress hormone that might join the mix and cause even more difficulties during the menopause. I will finish off by discussing how you can do your best to reduce the amount of stress you have in your life.

You must learn to handle stress healthily. Enough is going on in your life as things stand; you do not need extra worry and problems.

So, first things first, let's talk about what stress is.

Fight or Flight? The Dangers of Stress and the Role of Cortisol

Before I can explain why stress causes weight gain, I need to explain the stress process.

Stress is an emotion, but it is also a process and a reaction. To understand it, we need to go back to the days of cavemen and cavewomen. In that era, there were a million and one things to run away from. These included terrifying beasts who were trying to eat them. Of course, we do not have these problems to worry about nowadays, thankfully, but the human brain has not evolved since then on the stress front. I am talking about the "fight or flight" response here.

In those days, our ancestors would experience a fight or flight reaction to either turn towards the threat and fight it or run away from it. Those were the only two options.

The human brain is always on the lookout for a threat; something that is going to threaten our safety and well-being. That is why humans are hard-wired to be negative before they are positive; the brain is on safety mode most of the time.

So, while your brain is trying to keep you safe, it also perceives situations to be threatening when, in reality, they are not. When the brain decides that something is a threat, it kickstarts the stress process and gets the body ready to either fight it or run away from it. Extra endorphins are released to help you out in this situation, additional oxygen is available and a stress hormone cortisol is released.

Let's look at two examples now. In case number one, you face a real threatening situation. For example, a dangerous animal is about to attack you. What will you do? There are two options — you will run away from the threat or fight it and win, and the whole thing will be over. You will be affected by this and feel tired for a short while, but then you will be fine. Your hormonal levels will return to normal and your body will stop pumping out cortisol until the next time the brain recognises a threat.

In the second example, there is no real threat, and the brain has got it wrong. You have not fought something or run away from anything, but the brain is scanning the environment —worrying — and remains stuck in the stress zone. What does this mean? It means your body is on high alert and the cortisol is running loose around your body. You see, this is the situation we find ourselves in most of the time. We are sometimes late for an important meeting, worried about paying bills, going through a divorce, etc. These situations can cause stress, and our body will react to each of them as if we are facing a real danger.

When left to run wild in this situation, stress is damaging. In the first example, we face a real dangerous situation, and our body reacts to it accordingly. That is perfectly fine. It is what the body is supposed to do. However, the second example is not healthy. Unfortunately, it is a situation that is all too common in the fast-paced and demanding world we live in today.

So, what do high levels of cortisol do that is so damaging? The answer is — many things, but in the context of this book, it makes you put on weight. Several studies suggest that chronically raised cortisol levels contribute to increased insulin in the blood. This is one of the main contributors to weight gain as insulin controls the blood glucose level, which converts food energy into fat. We must not ignore the fact that raised cortisol level often causes cravings for sweets, high-fat and salty foods. Apart from contributing to the elevated insulin levels, these foods are also known to lead to poor health, low energy levels, and weight gain.

It is important to mention that when entering the perimenopausal stage, the decreased level of oestrogen tends to increase the cortisol level. Therefore, it is even more important to follow some basic self-care principles which include a plant-based diet and a healthy lifestyle. Your health and well-being depend on how much effort you put into taking proper care of your body.

As I have already mentioned, the menopause is a stressful time for many women and because you might experience its symptoms for anything up to 10 years, that is a long time for stress to be present in someone's body. While the lack of muscle mass can cause weight gain during this time, stress also adds to the situation and compounds it further.

As well as raising insulin, another reason for cortisol causing weight gain is that it stimulates the metabolism and demands from energy to come thick and fast. It is doing this because it is part of the stress reaction, i.e. the fight or flight response. It needs the energy to run or fight, even when there is nothing to fight with or run away from. In this situation, the body wants the energy quickly and tends to search for it from high-fat foods and carbs. A red light should be flashing straight away because those are two food groups that can certainly cause weight gain when used in the wrong way. And not only that but these foods are also damaging to your health. They cause inflammation in the body and can lead to serious diseases.

All of this stimulates the release of insulin, which then affects your overall blood sugar levels. Therefore, it is no surprise that a long period of stress can be a contributing risk factor for the development of diabetes over the long term. In effect, you will crave foods that are sweet, high in fat and therefore high in sugar and quite salty. These foods will cause you to pile on the pounds if you eat them too often, which you probably will if you are feeling too stressed over a more extended period.

So to conclude, cortisol is not your friend, and especially not during the menopause.

Why Is Stress so Common During the Menopause?

I have already mentioned this in passing, but let's discuss it further for clarity's sake.

I should point out that not every woman is going to feel stressed during the menopause. Some women do not feel stressed at all, others feel it occasionally and some women find their stress levels are continually high over this period. It is a personal experience that might differ from someone else's, but it is a time when you are more likely to notice issues and become more upset about them.

Many people struggle with changes in their lives, but it is hard to get away from it when the change is occurring within your body. This can cause anxiety. The more you sit and worry about it, the more stress is going to build up. If your menopausal symptoms are causing your lack of sleep, this is a significant precursor for stress once more.

You might also find that you are agitated and short tempered with your partner or the people around you. If this causes ructions within your relationships and friendships, you are again creating a stressful situation.

It is essential to mention that finding the right strategies to cope with stress in your life is as important as finding proper ways to manage stress inside your body. These two types of stress are closely connected and significantly affect one another. Their relationship impacts how you react to stressful situations you experience in life and any problem you face regularly.

There are countless reasons why the menopause might be a high-stress period for a woman, but the good news is that it is manageable when you educate yourself and learn how to change your mindset towards the positive. It is vital that you avoid unhealthy coping mechanisms, such as overeating, spending too much money on shopping treats, drinking too much alcohol, smoking, using drugs or spending countless hours watching Netflix. You need to focus your mind on healthy coping methods and as I will highlight in the next section, there are plenty of these that will help you deal with stress levels, but also aid your menopausal symptoms.

It is easy to say repeatedly that there is nothing to worry about concerning the menopause, that you are no less of a woman because of this process and that perhaps you are more of a woman because you have got your badge to prove it! However, if you are feeling confused, if you are struggling with specific symptoms, or you are just not having the best of times when it comes to the perimenopausal or menopausal period of your life, no amount of reassurances will make a difference. In this case, you need to get practical, and that is what I am going to talk about in this next section.

10 Stress Management Techniques to Try Today!

Finding ways to deal with stress will not magically make the menopause end, or get it over and done with, but will make the entire process easier and possibly make your life far more fulfilling and enjoyable to live as a result.

The good news is, stress management techniques are not too difficult, and anyone can do them. You simply need to choose the ones which work best for you. However, it is a good idea to give them all a try and figure it out from there — you never know what is going to work and what is not until you have tried it for yourself.

Let's check out the 10 stress management techniques that you can start today.

Talk About the Problem

You might not have a specific issue causing the stress, but you may generally be feeling stressed out. That is quite a common feeling for a woman going through the menopause because the whole situation feels out of control, or specific symptoms are too troublesome. In that case, find someone you trust, perhaps someone who is also going through the menopause or has already gone through it, and talk about it. Talking to a qualified counsellor is always a good option. A counsellor can help you find your unique way of expressing your feelings and managing your emotions about the situation you are currently facing.

It does not matter what you say to the person you chose to share your worries and concerns. Whether it is a trusted friend or a counsellor, tell them whatever comes into your mind. Just get it out there. Talk about how you feel, the things that worry you, and the nagging doubts in the back of your mind.

The more you empty your brain of things which are concerning you, the lighter you will feel. Most people find that when they talk about something, it helps put it into perspective. Offloading your thoughts and feelings can be incredibly cathartic. Seeing a counsellor and finding your voice can help you to see and feel about things differently. It can take the burden off your shoulders and bring positivity into your life.

If you are struggling with your weight loss or feeling upset about the weight gain, talk about it with someone you trust and perhaps put a weight loss plan together. Find a friend you can exercise with or join a class; this is motivating and will give your workout a social element.

Spend More Time Outdoors

Mother Nature perhaps is not treating you very well right now, but she also has lots of natural healing to send your way too — head outside! Sunlight and fresh air can help to reduce stress, anxiety and depression, allowing you to feel more uplifted and lighter on your feet.

When you are feeling low or worried about something, a short time breathing in the fresh air outside can help to distract you and take your worries away. You are also benefiting from the increased vitamin D from the sunlight which is linked to increased mood; a lack of vitamin D during the winter months is associated with low mood.

Serotonin is another naturally occurring hormone within the body. It has positive effects. It regulates your mood and helps with sleep, memory and feelings of happiness. Being outdoors and in the sunlight can boost your serotonin levels. This can help to achieve a more upbeat mood which, as a result, decreases your stress levels.

Get Plenty of Exercise

This particular stress management technique is ideal for menopausal weight gain problems because it helps to battle that specific issue, alongside a healthy diet.

Exercise has many benefits. It can support your weight loss as well as help you feel less stressed. Exercising is known to boost the mood and distract the mind. Working out is excellent stress relief. During exercise, the body produces endorphins in the brain. These chemicals act as natural painkillers, support your well-being, and help with sleep.

You can choose any exercise you like, but some are incredibly helpful for protecting the body against potential bone density loss, which contributes to osteoporosis in women over the menopausal age.

Try activities such as swimming, yoga or Pilates, as these are strength-building exercises which are also very low impact and easy to do. They help with breathing and this can reduce stress levels and improve sleep. Pilates moves are excellent for stretching and this helps with flexibility and balance. Swimming is perfect because you are surrounded by water, which is naturally calming. Yoga is another excellent choice because it teaches you to focus on your breathing and that in itself can help you overcome stressful situations when they occur.

Meditate and Try Mindfulness

Many women find meditation very useful when they feel stressed out, so this is certainly something you could try. The downside is that many women also struggle with meditation and give up too soon — this is something that takes time and practice, but the benefits are far-reaching once it is mastered. Quietening the mind can be difficult when there is so much going on, but it is possible with practice.

Try this:

- Choose a time when you will not be disturbed; turn your phone off and close the curtains.

- Sit or lay down somewhere comfortable.

- Close your eyes and turn your attention to your breathing.

- Breathe in slowly and steadily through your nose for the count of five.

- Hold the breath for a count of three.

- Slowly exhale through your mouth for a count of five.

- Repeat until you feel calm.

- If any thoughts try to enter your mind, simply acknowledge them and push them away.

- Keep focusing on your breathing until you have successfully managed to quieten the noise in your mind.

- Try and build up the amount of time you stay in the meditation exercise as you go along, but do not rush it.

- When you are ready, tell yourself that you are going to open your eyes and slowly do so, staying seated or laid down for a few minutes until you are feeling more alert.

You can try countless meditation types, but many women find guided group meditations to be very useful. You could seek out groups of women who are also going through this time in their lives and join in. This will allow you to meet new friends in the same situation as you and help banish your stress at the same time.

Something else you can try is mindfulness. This can be particularly useful when dealing with life changes that are the very crux of your stress. Mindfulness teaches you to live in the present moment and not to worry about the past or think too far into the future. That is something all of us could do with trying more!

Many women tend to think back over the past and their fertile years, perhaps comparing how they looked and felt back then to how they look and feel after menopausal weight gain. Being overweight can cause some women to feel unattractive. Also, excess weight can negatively impact our health and energy levels. It can be very easy to look back and make yourself feel bad about these changes. Similarly, you might be thinking too far into the future, worrying about what comes next and how you are going to deal with becoming a little older.

Using mindfulness can help push all of this to one side and help you to focus on you in the here and now. Also, meditation, reading inspiring books, and having regular contact with people who lift your spirit can significantly increase your confidence and improve the way you feel about yourself.

Again, it can be hard to do but you need to stick with it and practice, without trying to rush things. An excellent way to start is to head outside for a walk. Leave your phone at home or keep it on silent in your bag, and make sure that your attention is firmly on the place you are in right now, e.g. the road, the field, the park, the beach, or wherever else you are. Be in the here and now. Enjoy the moment!

Walk along at a slow pace if you can, and try the breathing exercise I mentioned a few paragraphs ago. Of course, keep your eyes open! Once you are calm enough, turn your attention to your surroundings. Notice the vibrant green of the leaves on the tree; really tune into them and notice how the sunlight glints off them, or how the wind gently blows them around.

Once you have taken in every element of that tree, slowly, turn your attention to something else, perhaps the clouds in the sky or the dog running around in the field next to you.

By being absorbed in the current moment, you keep your mind in the here and now, distracting yourself from unhelpful and stressful thoughts. Over time, you are going to notice a greater appreciation of what is around you and will not be bothered by petty worries half as much as you used to be. This is ideal for stress management, but it is also a great way to live.

Focus on Your Sleep

Focusing on your sleep is the key. It has such a powerful effect on your health and quality of life. Lack of sleep can be one of the menopausal symptoms and having problems with sleep can worsen stress. Therefore, focusing on improving the quality and duration of sleep is vital.

Easier said than done, yes, but totally possible.

If you are regularly struggling with sleep and feel you might have insomnia, it is a good idea to consult your doctor and see if anything can be done about this issue. However, most of the time, making some simple changes to your sleeping routine and implementing a few useful tips can help you to have a better quality sleep.

I will not go into too much detail here, as I am going to cover a whole chapter on the connection between sleep and weight loss a little later on. For now, however, simply know that you need to focus on getting the best night's sleep possible on a regular basis to avoid stress and keep your weight steady and consistent. Of course, you will also feel far better in yourself if you are rested and alert, compared to feeling tired and agitated. It is very easy to allow worries and stress to overwhelm you when you feel this way.

Remember, good quality sleep is a very powerful medicine. And it is one of the best habits to implement in your everyday life to achieve good health and successful weight loss, in addition to a healthy diet and regular exercise.

Focus on Your Enjoyment

What do you like to do in your spare time? Whatever it is, do more of it!

It is very easy to focus your time on everyone and everything else: work, family, children, friends — a long to-do list, and most women do not spend enough of their time on themselves. It is not selfish to focus on yourself occasionally. It is actually necessary for your overall health and well-being, and extremely useful for excluding stress from the equation.

If you love to lay in a bath and read a book, do it. If you like to go shopping with a friend, go for it, as long as you are not spending money to mask your emotional upset, of course. If you enjoy crafts, baking, cooking, playing sports, pampering yourself, or simply sitting and watching the world go by, you have permission to do it. It is necessary and it is advisable.

Be Sociable and Do not Hide Yourself Away

When you are not feeling your best self or perhaps feeling a little low about how you look (just because you have gained a few pounds) and stressed out about everything around you, menopause included, it is easy to hide away and avoid social situations. I advise you not to do this!

Get out there, live your life, focus on having fun and you will find that stress quickly leaves your life as a result. You will also find the confidence within yourself to handle whatever the menopause has thrown at you. If you are going out with friends in the same age group as you, it is likely they are going to be experiencing the same or similar issues as you. I remember having long conversations with female friends about how menopausal symptoms affected our lives. Oh, I so wish I knew back then what I know about coping mechanisms now.

Being involved in the conversation on the topic of menopause with other women can sometimes lead to plenty of laughter. Sharing the misery of the menopause usually creates a light-hearted atmosphere and can put women in a much better mood. *A problem shared is a problem halved*, they say. So, if you can find someone who can relate to your problem, it lightens the mood.

Try Visualisation

Many women find visualisation a useful tool for stress management, but it can be used for several other problems too, such as negative thinking or simply when you need the motivation to get something done. If you feel stressed out, worried, or just focused on the negative side of things, turn your attention to how you want something to work out. This is a time when you *are* allowed to think of the future because you are doing it through positive eyes and not worried ones.

Sit somewhere quiet and close your eyes. Focus on your breathing until you have calmed your mind. When you are ready, picture how you want things to look, for instance, how you want to feel and how you want your future life to be. The more you picture it and add in details, the more real and effective it will be when you call the picture to your mind during a period of stress.

Of course, make sure that the picture you are visualising is realistic. It will not help if you picture yourself as a size zero on a beach in two months; if you are overweight right now, this is simply not realistic and probably not something that will make you truly happy anyway. It is far better to focus yourself on being happy, healthy and body confident.

Visualisation will help you take actionable steps and pull you towards transformation with a much more powerful force.

Try Reframing Your Thoughts to Become More Positive

Stress happens far more readily when your mindset is generally negative. You may be feeling low because you are not happy with your appearance or struggling with menopausal symptoms. In this case, you need to try and focus on becoming more positive overall. By doing that, you will notice that your stress reduces, you have a new-found strength to overcome difficult emotions and you are able to look at life with a glass-half-full mentality.

Of course, changing your mindset in this way is not easy and may take a while to complete the process. Despite this, it is a very worthwhile way to spend your time.

Reframing is a cognitive behaviour therapy treatment method that seeks to change a person's mindset from negative to positive and can help with a wide range of different problems.

There is no reason why you cannot use it in this situation.

The downside of reframing is that you need to be continually aware of your thoughts at the start, and that is pretty tiring and time-consuming. Again, it is worthwhile. Stress will find it harder to overtake your life if you think more positively.

Try this:

- The next time you recognise that you are thinking something negative, acknowledge it as being negative.

- Think of something positive to counteract that negative thought. For instance, if you are thinking "My body is changing and I do not like it", change it to "How my body changes make me understand its power". You can use any example you want; this is just one of them.

- Then, repeat the positive thought several times, and try your best to visualise it too. If you can, say it aloud, as this will be more powerful and more useful to you.

- Repeat this with every negative thought you recognise.

Focus on Your Diet

We will dedicate a whole chapter to diet in a short while, so I will not dwell on the finer details here. However, when you are eating healthily — feeding your body with the right amounts of carbs, protein and fat, and getting all the vitamins and minerals you need — you can manage your weight more effectively as a result. You are going to be more upbeat and confident in yourself. That is a picture which stress will find difficult to creep into. We can compare this to putting the correct type of fuel into your car. If you fill the tank with the wrong fuel, it might damage your engine, and your vehicle will not be going anywhere.

When you feel stressed, you are also more likely to reach for unhealthy food choices as a way of coping. You know how it goes: you say to yourself, "I deserve a slice of chocolate cake, I have been so stressed out lately", but one slice leads to two or three, and then you start beating yourself up internally for not being more careful with your food choices.

Of course, those slices of chocolate cake usually go straight to your hips, and as I have mentioned already, menopausal weight gain is far harder to lose *now* than previously.

And no, this does not mean you cannot have the odd treat, or that you have to deny yourself everything you enjoy. It is all about moderation. That is key to achieving success with your health and weight loss goals, and we are going to look at it in the following chapter.

Key Points

This chapter has talked about the dangers of stress and how the menopause can be an incredibly stressful time for women. When left unchecked and allowed to grow, stress can be fatal. However, stress is something we all deal with in small amounts. Learning to handle stress by using stress management techniques is a vital part of the whole menopausal process. By mastering these, you will find that your menopausal story is far more comfortable to manage as a result.

The main points to remember from this chapter are:

- Stress can be extremely damaging to health when allowed to build up and remain in place for an extended period.

- The menopause can cause stress to a woman simply because her hormones are running wild, or she might be struggling to deal with the symptoms in general.

- The stress process is often referred to as "fight or flight".

- Much of the time, the brain misjudges what a real threat is, and as a result, the stress process kickstarts for no reason.

- During the stress reaction, the body releases a cortisol hormone, which can lead to weight gain over time.

- Learning to handle stress will allow you to be healthier, happier, and help you control your weight more successfully.

Chapter 4

Healthy Diet 101

Handling stress and approaching the menopause with a positive mindset is only part of the deal. Hormones may stimulate weight gain, but the food you put into your body will most likely cause you to gain weight at the end of the day.

The hormones might cause you to feel hungrier and make you less firm to resist food cravings, but if you are putting healthy foods into your body and focus on quality, you are far less likely to put weight on even if you consume more food than you require.

But do you know what a healthy diet is?

Many people falsely believe that a healthy diet means restriction and not being able to eat what you want. In truth, that is a fad diet and those types of diets do not work! If you are always on a fad diet, you will probably end up eating more in the end because the foods you eat will not satisfy you, and you will be fed up with not enjoying your favourite foods now and again, so you will rebel against it.

In this chapter, I am going to talk about what a healthy diet is, and what it is not. Of course, even if you stick to healthy food options and avoid going towards the unhealthier ones, you will still have to occasionally battle with your hormones, but remember one word throughout it all — moderation.

Moderation is key!

That means you can enjoy the odd slice of pizza, the occasional bar of chocolate, or the occasional glass of wine and it is totally fine and even encouraged, as long as the rest of your diet is healthy. Besides a nutritious diet, you should also make sure that you exercise regularly, but we will go over that in more detail shortly. Focusing on what is right for your body 80% of the time is all you need to do.

Remember, a healthy diet needs to be part of your lifestyle and not something you only do for a short while. If you want to avoid and rectify menopausal weight gain, you need to dedicate time to making life changes. So, in this case, moderation is going to be the one thing that you must apply to your new lifestyle. This will prevent you from making it so difficult for yourself that it is impossible to stay on track.

What does moderation look like?

It means you have a slice of pizza when you fancy and not the whole pizza. You have a glass of wine instead of the entire bottle, and you only have it once or twice a week. Even if you want alcoholic drinks every night, choose which two days you want to have them, and you stick to your decision. You have a few squares of chocolate rather than devouring a family-sized bar, or you have a takeaway once a week and not every night.

Moderation means you have a little of what you want, but in ways which mean it does not ruin your entire healthy lifestyle outlook.

You Really are What You Eat

We have all heard the saying, *You are what you eat*. This is true in so many ways and I agree to it. If you regularly eat processed meals and sugary snacks, and load up on sugary drinks every day, you will notice that your health suffers.

Your health and weight will be affected by unhealthy eating and poor drinking habits.

Your skin will break out, your hair will lack shine, perhaps you will feel tired and sluggish, your sleep might be affected at night due to indigestion or the blood sugar crash, and of course, you are going to notice your clothes becoming a little tighter.

On the other hand, if you eat a healthy diet, you are healthier on the inside, and it shows on the outside. Your skin will glow, your hair will shine, your nails will be stronger and you will have more energy. You will be positive as a result of how you feel, and you will notice that you not only lose weight, but you maintain your ideal weight once you hit it. Your clothes will fit better, you will feel lighter on your feet and overall, you will simply feel more confident as a result of the physical effects.

So, if you eat poorly, you are unhealthy. If you eat well, you are healthy.

The foods you eat determine how healthy your body is going to be.

The problem with menopausal weight gain is that it can happen quickly and without warning. If your diet is not healthy to begin with, you are going to find that shifting the excess weight is an uphill battle. If you are eating healthily to start with, you might have the cravings that your hormonal imbalances cause, but if you have the right mindset, you will not have a major problem to deal with because you will not be reaching for unhealthy food choices.

The bottom line is that menopausal weight gain comes down to the ability to handle temptation. Your hormones are going to make you want to eat and they are going to turn their attention towards the worst types of foods. The hunger hormone is on the rampage and the satiety hormone, which responsibility is to reduce your appetite, has somehow disappeared. Giving in makes you feel worse in yourself, so you just eat more to make yourself feel better. It is such a vicious circle that so many women fall foul of, and before they realise it, they are faced with weight gain which takes a tremendous amount of effort to lose.

Hormones are potent, and you should never underestimate their ability to make you want to eat everything in the fridge or kitchen cupboards. You should also never underestimate how overwhelming the cravings can be. However, if you are hooked on the right types of food, the damage will be minimal, if at all.

So, while you are what you eat, if what you are eating is healthy, you do not have so much of a problem to begin with.

The Key Nutrients You Need Daily

During the menopause, as we have already explored, oestrogen and progesterone levels begin to decline. This can detrimentally affect your metabolism. It is important to ensure that your diet is therefore focused on health and well-being rather than towards enjoyment of all the processed and sugary foods the world likes to throw at us.

A healthy diet consists of macronutrients and micronutrients.

Macronutrients include:

- Protein

- Carbohydrate

- Fat

Micronutrients include:

- Vitamins

- Minerals

Do not be afraid to eat fats; simply make sure that you opt for the healthier versions. You need to look towards monounsaturated and polyunsaturated fats as a rule of thumb. Avoid trans fat as much as possible. This type of fat damages your health and causes weight gain.

Apart from macronutrients, you also need a range of different micronutrients, such as magnesium, potassium, zinc, iron, calcium and vitamins (A, B, C, D, E, etc.). These are important for the optimal health of your body.

To keep your body healthy, stick to eating whole organic foods as often as possible. These foods store beneficial nutrients that give your body energy and help to support and ensure the functioning of your main organs. Weight gain is a complicated process and can be put down to a range of different causes. When you feed your body with healthy foods and focus on portion sizes — not too much and not too little — you have a chance of maintaining a healthy weight. Of course, it is also essential to pay attention to your lifestyle and make sure you focus on implementing healthy choices as much as you can.

To ensure that your body receives all the essential nutrients needed for its healthy functioning, you should get the majority of your calories from foods such as fresh fruits and fresh vegetables, legumes, protein (lean), nuts and whole grains. When you consume too many foods or beverages that are high in trans fat and calories, e.g. fizzy drinks, chocolate or ice cream, you are not doing your body any favours and it is a recipe for weight gain!

The problem is, when your hormones are playing havoc with your metabolism, your body is automatically going to start craving the foods and drinks which are high in fat and sugar. Those foods can be detrimental to your health.

There are different types of diets. Some of them are focused mainly on counting calories. Others involve fasting and focusing on restricting daily eating windows. The popular Keto diet tends to be more focused on cutting back on carbs and increasing fats' consumption. In this book, I am not promoting any particular diet; I just want to outline a healthy diet as simply as possible to help you understand what you should be aiming for, versus what you should not. Understanding what a healthy diet includes and what your body requires, will help you decide what type of diet is the best for you.

Remember, here you are looking for a healthy lifestyle for the rest of your life, so it needs to be simple, flexible, and easy to follow, allowing you some "wiggle" room whenever you fancy something on the naughty list. If the food is high in calories or trans fats, it does not mean you can never eat it, it simply means that you need to adopt the moderation rule I mentioned earlier.

Many different types of food are ideal for menopause-aged women, since they contain micronutrients that can help overcome some of the negative effects of this time of life. For instance, magnesium is shown to help with bone mass and improve sleep; therefore, it is essential for menopausal women to include magnesium in their diet. This mineral is found in green leafy vegetables as well as in many fruits, nuts and seeds. In addition, vitamin C is essential for maintaining the health of your hair when you may be experiencing hair loss or thinning. This is one of the common menopausal symptoms and therefore it is advisable to consume foods rich in vitamin C, such as citrus fruits. Some women use vitamin C in the form of a supplement, but we will deal with this subject later.

Macronutrients are also known to provide your body with different benefits. For instance, carbohydrates will give you energy when you are feeling tired, and protein will help you feel fuller for longer, meaning you are less likely to give in to cravings or turn to unhealthy food options. Protein makes enzymes and hormones and is a building block of your muscle, skin and blood. Regarding fats, choosing to eat healthy types will help you lower the chances of heart disease and stroke. Healthy fats in your diet will rebuild your cells and stabilise your hormones.

You can see now how eating various foods, rather than relying on limited types, provides your body with everything it needs for healthy functioning and longevity.

Let's look in more detail at the types of foods you should be eating to help with your weight loss and other menopausal symptoms, and ensure that you follow a healthy diet in general.

Dairy Products

Dairy contains calcium, magnesium, phosphorus and vitamins K and D. These are all ideal vitamins to ensure bone health and strength. As you are probably aware, there is a chance of osteoporosis in later life if your bone density levels become too low due to a lack of oestrogen. This issue is particularly common with menopausal women. Consuming a substantial amount of dairy in the diet can help to prevent bone problems.

There is also a suggestion that dairy products may help to contribute towards a better night's sleep. This is because of the tryptophan found in dairy, which helps induce sleep. We have already talked about the fact that sleep can be affected during the menopausal period. A little later, I am going to talk in much more detail about sleep and how you can do your best to ensure that you are getting enough of it.

Healthy Fats, i.e. The Good Guys

When you hear the word "fat" you probably automatically think of the negative connotation, but the body needs a certain amount of fat in order to thrive.

There are good types of fat and there are bad ones too. Avoid the bad guys, such as trans fats, commonly found in processed meals, fried foods, and high-fat dairy products. Instead, focus on polyunsaturated fats, monounsaturated fats and omega 3 fatty acids.

Omega 3 fatty acids are commonly found in oily types of fish, such as salmon, anchovies and mackerel. If you are not a fish fan, you can also find them in some seeds, such as flax, hemp, chia, walnuts, pine nuts, and Brazil nuts in small amounts.

Of course, if you feel you are not getting enough Omega 3 through your food, then using a supplement, such as fish oil, might be a good option for you. It is essential to check out any supplements you consider taking with your doctor before you go ahead. It is common for supplements to interfere with any prescribed medication. For this reason, I strongly advise you to consult a medical practitioner about your intentions, to avoid any adverse effects of drug interactions that could damage your health.

Healthy types of fat not only help to regulate your weight and maintain satiety, reduce cravings for the harmful fats, but they may also reduce the severity of your hot flushes and night sweats. Again, this could help you get a better night's sleep if night sweats create a problem for you.

Primary sources of healthy fats include:

- Avocado

- Oily types of fish

- Olives

- Unsalted versions of nuts, cashew nuts, peanuts and almonds

- Oils made from seeds or plants, including extra-virgin olive oil, coconut oil, avocado oil, peanut oil, sesame oil, soybean oil, etc.

Eating healthy fat is necessary for your health. It provides your body with energy, protects you against heart disease, and helps your cells grow. Healthy fats can also support your weight loss by controlling your blood sugar levels and suppressing your appetite.

Wholegrains

The benefit of wholegrains for anyone trying to lose weight is that they are filling. This means you are less likely to snack on unhealthy options and are less likely to crave sugar and other unhealthy foods. Wholegrains are also high in fibre and vitamin B, which can benefit your overall health. Your body digests fibre more slowly than simple carbohydrates like starch and sugar, so the fibre from wholegrains keeps you feeling full for a more extended period.

We are all advised to eat wholegrains, regardless of age, because they offer many health benefits. When eaten as part of a balanced diet, they can protect against heart disease, diabetes and some types of cancer. The fact that wholegrains can keep you fuller for longer is a great way to deal with cravings and menopausal weight gain.

The types of foods to be on the lookout for include brown rice, rye, quinoa and barley.

Fresh Fruit and Vegetables

Everyone needs to get the right amount of fresh fruit and vegetables in their diet, regardless of gender or age. This used to be five a day, but then it went up to seven a day, and then there was some mention of 10. My advice? Do not bother trying to hit targets, just make sure that you pack your daily diet with plenty of fresh fruit and vegetables and you are good to go. There is no need to complicate matters further.

These products are brimming with a vast range of different vitamins and minerals and plenty of highly powerful antioxidants. These can keep you in optimum health and also keep your immune system strong. It has been shown that plenty of fresh fruit and vegetables, and fibre, may help postmenopausal women reduce the number of hot flushes and night sweats they experience.

If you want to know more about what you can do about those symptoms, I recommend you to have a look at my book *Free Yourself From Hot Flushes and Night Sweats: The Essential Guide to a Happy and Healthy Menopause*, which is available on Amazon.

Try and get the right amount of cruciferous vegetables into your diet too. This includes broccoli, cauliflower, kale, Brussels sprouts, cabbage and bok choy, to name a few, as well as colourful berries for powerful antioxidants.

Protein

Lean protein is vital for your overall health and well-being and is one of the main macronutrients that helps your body thrive. Consuming an adequate amount of protein ensures the healthy functioning of your body and contributes to bone health.

Remember, during the menopause, oestrogen declines, which is linked to decreased muscle mass, slowing down your metabolism and increasing the potential for lack of bone strength. Protein is required to protect against all of this.

The general guidelines are that menopausal women, over the age of 50 in particular, should eat 0.45-0.55 grams of lean protein per pound of their body weight. This is equal to 1-1.5 grams of lean protein per kilogram of their body weight. This averages out to around 20-25 grams of protein per meal if you weigh 10 stone or 63.5 kilograms.

For example, two eggs have around 26 grams of protein, and one steak has approximately 20 grams of protein.

You can also find a large quantity of protein in green leafy vegetables. This shows it is not so hard to meet your daily body needs and ensure you eat the right amount of protein.

To get a good amount of protein in your diet, you should look towards lean meat, fish, dairy products, eggs and legumes.

Water

Water is the most important nutrient that you can give to your body, whatever your age. Most of your body is made of water, and you keep losing it through sweating, breathing, urinating, etc. We even lose water while we sleep, and every milliliter of water needs to be replenished. Remember that the more you exercise, the more water you will need to drink. You also require more water if you live in a hot climate. I encourage you always to carry a water bottle. It will help you to stay hydrated.

Some of the benefits of drinking water include:

- Flushing out toxins

- Helping with digestion

- Regulating your body temperature

- Helping to prevent constipation

- Increasing energy

- Helping with weight loss

- Lubricating the joints

In my book, *Live Healthy on a Tight Schedule*, there is a section focusing on how to drink more water. Here are the key points of this section:

- Reports show that women should drink approximately 2.7 litres of water per day.

- Hydration can come from various sources, and some foods can be a good source of water.

- Foods that are very high in water content include various fruit and vegetables such as cucumbers, tomatoes, spinach, melon, oranges, broccoli, and berries.

- Consuming foods with a high water content not only helps you stay hydrated, but also provides you with fibre and various vitamins and minerals, all playing an essential role in keeping your body healthy.

- Drinking water needs to become a habit. Start by keeping a log of each time you drink water during the day, and estimate how much you have consumed.

Learn to appreciate water; it is the healthiest drink of them all.

Foods Which Contain Phytoestrogens

Certain types of food contain something called phytoestrogens. Now, anything with the word "oestrogen" in it should shout out to you as being useful for a menopausal woman, who suddenly finds herself lacking in this all-important hormone.

Phytoestrogens are found in some plants and act as a weak type of oestrogen which is in compound form. These are not the same as the hormone that declines in your body during the menopause, but they may help you deal with some particular symptoms, such as hot flushes. These types of foods are also healthy, so by packing these into your diet, you are also ensuring that you are on the right side of the health spectrum and you are doing your best to stay away from that pesky menopausal weight gain problem.

You may want to consider taking supplement called *Isoflavone* to reduce your menopausal symptoms. If this is the case, I suggest you ALWAYS check with your doctor if it safe for you to take it.

For naturally occurring phytoestrogens, look towards foods such as soy and red clover. The general advice is, if your diet is plant-based and is very rich in a variety of fruits, vegetables, legumes and some grains, then you are most likely consuming the necessary amounts of phytoestrogens through the food you eat.

So, now you know about the types of foods that are helpful for menopausal women, which will help you be healthy and avoid weight gain during this time in your life and in the future.

Now, let's look at which foods should you avoid?

This part is fairly easy and is the general advice that you would give anyone of any age if they have decided to become healthier and lose weight. However, certain foods may aggravate menopausal symptoms; you need to eliminate these for the time being to give you a more comfortable menopausal experience.

In general, you should avoid:

- **Foods containing added sugar** – Foods that may affect your blood sugar levels have been linked to an increase in hot flushes. A little later, we will talk about the role of blood sugar in weight gain, but for now, know that any foods that have added sugars are very unhealthy and not useful if you are struggling with hot flushes already. Sugar is linked to weight gain and increases the risks of diabetes, stroke and heart disease.

- *Processed carbohydrates* – Try and steer clear of baked goods (you can do it!) and white bread. These can increase your blood sugar levels and therefore contribute to hot flushes, while also being seriously bad for your waistline.

- *Alcohol* – Remember that watching what you drink is vital to controlling your weight. In addition to affecting your weight, alcohol prevents your body from absorbing vitamins and minerals. Therefore, alcoholic drinks are likely to have a significant impact on your overall health. Most alcoholic beverages are high in sugar, which will not help you battle your weight gain or control hot flushes. Remember, if you want a glass of wine or any other alcoholic beverage, do so in moderation. It is recommended that a menopausal woman should drink no more than one drink a day, which is equivalent to having seven drinks a week.

- *Spicy foods* – We are often told that eating spicy foods can be useful for weight loss because they help boost metabolism in some cases, but in terms of the menopause, the spice factor could make hot flushes worse.

- **Too much salt** – Excess amount of salt in food is not a healthy option for anyone. For a menopausal woman, it may lower your bone density over time, which could contribute to your chances of developing osteoporosis. Of course, the decrease in oestrogen also causes problems for your general health and your bones' health, but you can reduce this risk by reducing the amount of salt you eat.

Eating a healthy diet is not difficult in theory, but in practice, when you have got a million cravings coming your way and have never really tried to eat healthily before, it can be difficult. For the most part, you can find all the nutrients your body needs from the foods you eat, but in some cases, you may be tempted towards taking a supplement to improve your overall health or to manage some health conditions.

Before you take any type of supplement, be sure to consult your doctor. For the most part, many supplements are fine to take, but everyone's physiology is slightly different, therefore they will affect your health differently. I suggest you clear things with your doctor before beginning to use any supplement. This especially applies to you if you are taking any prescribed medication. Mixing supplements with certain medicines can be hazardous. Therefore, you must talk to your doctor about this.

Your doctor might recommends following supplements:

- Iron

- Evening primrose oil

- Potassium

- Magnesium

- Zinc

- Calcium

- Omega 3 fatty acids

- Vitamin A

- B vitamins, including B2, B6, B9 and B12

- Vitamin C

- Vitamin D

- Vitamin E

This is not an exhaustive list of the supplements your doctor may suggest you take. It will depend upon your health, diet, and current and past medical history.

Why Fad Diets do not Work

The last section was a lengthy one, but I hope that it crushed some myths about healthy eating and that you can now see that it is not particularly challenging to follow a healthy diet. You simply need to make healthy food choices. The more you do it, the more you will find yourself pulling away from unhealthy options, because you feel so great in yourself that you do not want to ruin it! You will also find that you can summon up the willpower to avoid giving in to cravings.

There are many ways you can meet your daily nutritional needs but following a fad diet is certainly not one of them. You should never go down the route of a fad diet. This type of diet is the one that does not support your health and it only focuses on weight loss. Fad diets do not strive to feed your body with quality foods such as organic fruit and vegetables or grass-fed meat for example, but instead they focus entirely on losing a few extra pounds in weight. Following a fad diet is not a sustainable way to live.

However, if you stick to a healthy, balanced diet, you will find that you are getting the right amount of nutrients, which is essential to your overall well-being.

I have mentioned the word "fad" a few times, and I want to explore this a little more before we move on.

I cannot stress enough that fad diets are not healthy. The companies and individuals behind these diets will tell you that they have discovered the quick route towards losing weight and that you will be in your bikini by the end of next week. They are lying! It is not possible to lose weight quickly and keep it off, not without severely damaging your health and making you miserable.

Any diet that involves counting points, advising you to stop consuming all kind of fat, permitting you to eat sugary and other unhealthy foods as long as you stick to your calorie allowance, or following theories that negatively impact your health, needs to go out the window. Keep it simple, and just choose healthy options over unhealthy ones. It is not rocket science. It works, but only if you commit to it.

Become food label savvy and understand that it is not good to eat it if the food is high in the wrong types of fat. Learn to grill, bake, or griddle your food rather than fry it and opt for healthy oils rather than unhealthy options. Snack on fruits and vegetables or nuts and seeds, rather than chocolate and ice cream, and know that there are hidden sugars in many drinks which claim to be "diet" or "zero calorie" versions. Water is always better and if you find it too bland, add a quick squeeze of fresh lemon or lime. Your body will benefit from the high level of vitamin C from these fruits.

Of course, the most important thing you should remember is that "M" word once again – moderation. Fad diets do not allow you to have anything you enjoy without ruining your hard work. If you crave a slice of pizza and follow a fad diet, you have zero chance of it being allowed. You will then have it anyway and feel bad that you have "ruined" your diet. This often leads to a binge session of all the foods you have missed so badly, which will make you feel much worse, telling yourself that you are a dietary failure and beat yourself up about it for weeks afterwards.

That is the damaging cycle of a fad diet.

I would like to remind you to visit bit.ly/menopause-healthy-recipes-2 and download a free *Healthy Eating for Menopause – Recipe Book*. You will find simple and nutritious recipes that will support your health and weight loss goals.

When you eat healthily as much as possible, commit to moving your body more and enjoy your favourite foods in moderation, you are not restricting yourself to the point where you feel guilty for having a glass of wine or a few squares of chocolate. Life is too short to not feel the delicious melt of chocolate on your tongue or the zingy flavor of wine as it triggers your taste buds. Provided you do this in moderation, there is nothing to feel guilty about and no harm done. In some ways, it can even help you out, because it keeps your spirits up and ensures that you do not completely rebel against the new lifestyle you have chosen for yourself, which you intend to live for many years to come.

As you start to see results, you will feel so good about yourself that you will find it much easier to resist the cravings that your hormones might try and throw your way. This extra confidence will also help you to feel your best self as you go through the menopause. This is a time in life when many women feel less than their best, when they start to feel that they are getting older and perhaps missing out on the days of their youth. Of course, this is not the truth; menopause does not mean that anything is over, other than your periods – and for most women that is a good thing!

The more confident you are, the happier you are, the healthier you are, and the more able you are to deal with anything the menopause, or life in general, will throw at you. You will also find that it is much easier to lose weight because you are stuck on making healthy choices from this point onwards.

The Power of Journaling

Many women find it useful to keep a food journal. This works on many levels, but if you want to avoid making unhealthy food options, a food journal can show you where your trouble spots are and help put into place mechanisms to avoid falling foul of them in the future.

It is not unusual for your body to suddenly start to dislike a particular type of food or have a sensitivity or intolerance towards it, seemingly out of the blue. You might begin to notice stomach disturbances, bloating, or that you just do not feel your best after eating a specific ingredients. Keeping a food journal can help you identify this and then you can cut it out of your diet and see how that affects the way you feel.

Journaling is also an incredibly powerful tool for anyone trying to control their weight.

Invest in an attractive notebook and at the end of every day, write down what you ate for each meal, including drinks and snacks. Continue your journal for a couple of weeks in order to get a full picture of your eating habits.

Be sure to note down anything you felt was out of the ordinary too. For instance, if you ate a cheese sandwich on white bread and you felt bloated straight afterwards, write it down. Then, look for other occurrences when you experienced bloating after eating white bread. If you notice it more than once, try changing white bread to wholemeal and see if you notice a difference.

Journaling is a great way to get a total overview of your dietary picture. You might think you are eating healthily, but it is only when you see what you consume over a day in black and white that you might realise just how unhealthy your diet is. Some people do not know how much sugar they eat until they reflect back on it, and others perhaps do not realise how much salt or alcohol they consume. A journal can give you this information and therefore put the control of your diet into your hands.

Journaling is useful for anyone trying to lose weight or improve their general health. It can help you to understand more about the foods you are craving. In your journal, be sure to write down when you have cravings and what types of foods you were desperate for.

You might find that at a specific point in the day, over several days, you are craving sugar. This can be resolved by changing your eating habits a little and perhaps eating some healthy snacks before that trouble hotspot time. You can then reassess for a bit longer and see if the craving subsides due to your direct actions.

A journal is also a useful way to identify whether you may need to start taking supplements. Before a doctor advises you to take some supplements, they will ask you about your general diet and may ask you to keep a journal for a couple of weeks. This will provide them with evidence of what you are lacking and what you might have too much of. Your journal will help them to identify what your body needs.

What Is Your Magic Number?

If you find that you need to lose weight, you must aim for a realistic weight for you. Just because a particular celebrity is a size zero, it does not mean that you need to be. Just because your friend is a size 10, it does not mean you should be the same size. We all have a magic number, a weight at which we feel comfortable, healthy and happy.

Following advice from this book, you have a higher chance of reaching your healthy weight.

You will be able to identify your magic number quite easily as you start to lose weight; it is the number at which your body simply settles. This is the weight that gives you confidence. It is the weight at which you do not put on weight easily, but you do not lose it either. It is your body's happy weight at which you are healthy and feel good in yourself.

When you reach that number, assuming it is a healthy one and that your BMI is within the healthy range, stay there and do not attempt to lose a little more in order to fit into a smaller dress size. Simply learn how to maintain it. Nobody is worth more or less just because they fit into a size 6, 8, 10, or anything over or above. As long as you are healthy and happy, that is really all that matters.

Before we move on from the subject of what a healthy diet should look like, I do need to mention one final thing on this topic. I have already touched upon the idea that during the menopause, decreased levels of oestrogen and progesterone can cause a blood sugar imbalance which can affect your weight gain and cause you mood swings, lack of sleep, depression or anxiety. Blood sugar imbalance is also known to lead to developing heart disease, obesity, type 2 diabetes, Alzheimer's disease and other life-threatening conditions. For this reason, you must control your blood sugar levels, which you can achieve comfortably through a healthy diet and lifestyle.

"Blood sugar balancing" is a simple way of managing your weight and keeping your body healthy. Let me briefly explain the basic principles of a blood sugar balancing diet, what it is and what you can do about it.

It is important to mention that if your diet is already reasonably healthy, you will not need to implement many changes, but if your diet is not very healthy, then pay attention to what I am about to say.

This is how blood sugar balancing works. After eating a meal, the food is broken down and turned into glucose (sugar), which then enters your bloodstream. Certain foods create more glucose than others, in which case your body produces more insulin. The role of insulin is to remove the sugar from the blood, but the downside is that insulin is a fat-storage hormone and causes weight gain. The key is to know which food spikes the blood sugar levels so that you can eat less of it. You also need to find out which foods are safe to eat so you can eat more of them and have a lean and healthy body.

As a general rule, this is how to keep your blood sugar balance stable throughout the day:

- Base your meals on protein and healthy fats. These macronutrients will keep your blood sugar stable.

- Eat fibre-rich foods. This includes plenty of fruit and vegetables.

- Avoid foods with a high GI (glycemic index) rating and opt for foods with a low GI rating instead. Low GI foods include non-starchy vegetables such as lentils, green vegetables and green beans, while medium GI foods include oatmeal, sweet potatoes, peas and brown rice. Foods to avoid have a high GI and include white bread, white potatoes, white pasta, cakes, sweets, etc.

- Plan your meals ahead of time to ensure that you always have healthy foods at hand.

- Eat small meals more frequently throughout the day to avoid getting too hungry and then eating a large meal as this can spike your blood sugar levels.

- Take snacks out with you in your handbag or a car, so you are not tempted to opt for anything which could throw your blood sugar out of sync.

- Eat your breakfast. Make sure you avoid sugary cereals and start the day with a protein-based breakfast.

- Avoid sweetness or refined sugars and opt for natural sweeteners, such as honey or maple syrup, used in small amounts.

By keeping your blood sugar levels in check, you are contributing towards your overall health and well-being. This will help you reduce risk factors that could lead to serious health concerns. In addition to health risks, blood sugar imbalance can cause irritability, fatigue, headaches or food cravings, forcing you to turn to sugar-loaded carbohydrates, like pasta or bread, to gain energy.

My final advice in this chapter is to assess your weight and ask yourself the following question: do you need to lose weight because your current weight puts your health at risk? If so, make changes to your diet and lifestyle as described in this book to reduce your weight in a slow and steady manner. Fad diets might promise you a massive weight loss within a short period of time, but such an approach is totally unsustainable over the long term.

Make sure that you are working towards realistic targets and you are not trying to aim towards something that is completely out of reach, unsustainable or unhealthy. It is fine to be curvy, provided you are healthy on the inside. Equally, it is fine to be slim or skinny as long as you are healthy on the inside. There is no "one size fits all" answer here; it entirely depends on your body type, genetics, health, and ideal aim. Just make sure that whatever that aim is, it is realistic and achievable for you. I advise you to continue with your healthy lifestyle even after you have lost the weight. By doing this, you will be able to manage any possible weight gain as a result of the menopause.

Key Points

We have covered a lot of ground in this chapter. However, everything I have shared with you is super-useful and super-relevant to your health in general. There is never a negative side to being healthy; you really are what you eat and that means you need to be careful of what you are putting into your body if you want to look and feel your best.

We also know that the hormonal effects of the menopause have a nasty habit of causing weight gain if you are not clued up beforehand on what may happen. Far too many women are unaware that weight gain is a possible side effect of the menopause, and then they are shocked when they get on the scales or notice that their clothes are becoming tighter.

It is much harder to lose weight as you get older, simply because your metabolism is not as fast as it used to be. Keeping and maintaining a healthy weight during this time will make life easier for you, keep your confidence levels up and help you handle the effects of the menopause more comfortably and positively.

Here are the main points to take from this chapter:

- Health and well-being should be at the forefront of your mind at all times, ensuring that you battle any potential menopause weight gain before it begins.

- Vitamins and minerals that are essential to a menopausal woman include magnesium, calcium, B vitamins, etc. They can be consumed through a healthy diet or by taking supplements.

- Eating a balanced diet will ensure you get a range of macronutrients and micronutrients.

- Fad diets are to be avoided. Anything that is causing you to restrict your intake to significant levels is not necessary (unless a medical practitioner suggests it due to health reasons) and is likely to cause you to rebel against just how restrictive the diet is. Avoid at all costs!

- Moderation is key! You can have a little of what you fancy, even if it falls within the "bad for you" category, provided you pull back on other days and only have it occasionally and in a small amount.

- Changes to your diet have to be a lifestyle change and not something you only do for a few weeks.

- Always speak to a qualified person to get the best advice if you feel that you are not getting the optimal range of vitamins and minerals in your diet and also if you are looking at getting supplements.

- During the menopause, hormonal imbalance can cause blood sugar to become unstable. Therefore, you need to make sure that you consume a healthy diet, which includes eating little and often and avoiding any foods which are known to spike your blood sugar quickly, such as baked goods and high GI rated foods.

- If you need to lose weight, make sure that you are choosing a weight that is realistic for you and is not going to push you to painful and unhealthy limits.

Chapter 5

The Vital Role of Exercise

At any stage of life, you need to keep your body healthy and strong. This is especially important for women going through the menopause when all manner of changes occur. It is easy to put exercise to one side, assuming that we do not have time, or it is simply too hard. There are countless ways you can incorporate a little more movement into your day and therefore obtain the significant benefits of exercise.

You do not have to join the gym, or hire a personal trainer, or sweat it out every single day to become a healthier person; you simply need to eat healthily, ensure you are getting a range of vitamins and minerals, and move your body more. That is what exercise is, in its most simplistic form — it is moving your body more.

At this stage in your life, exercise is vital.

In this chapter, I will talk about the benefits of exercising and give you some ideas and inspiration regarding the best types of exercise for menopausal women. You will also learn how physical activity can easily fit into a healthy lifestyle.

Exercise does not have to be torture. It can be fun! Look at Zumba classes for a start — sure, they make you sweat, but they are great fun and help you make new friends too. My idea of fun is to go swimming and play tennis. I have a few more hobbies that I enjoy doing, but these two are very much part of my life and have been for years.

There is no downside when it comes to exercising regularly, but like everything else, you should not overdo it either. That is also something I want to talk about. You need to find the sweet spot — the amount of exercise that is healthy for you, giving you benefits and not making you feel exhausted and causing more problems than it is worth. What I am trying to say here is that pushing your body too hard through exercise might not bring the desired benefits, but instead it will be causing some damage.

The body of a menopausal woman needs the right type of exercise as much as it needs rest; otherwise, the combination of too much exercise and going through hormonal changes, are likely to cause stress and push your body to the limit. This might lead to adrenal fatigue, which is why finding the right exercise during this stage of your life is crucial.

The most common symptoms of adrenal fatigue include anxiety, having difficulties sleeping, craving sugary and salty foods, experiencing a lack of energy and reduced tolerance to stress.

We know that during the menopause weight gain is probable. We also know that menopausal women are at high risk of developing visceral fat around the middle and around the abdominal area. It has been proven that those are the hardest types of fat to lose. We also know that regular exercise will not only help prevent weight gain but also help lose the excess weight that you already carry. In addition, taking regular exercise that is right for your body will decrease the likelihood of having your weight creep back on after the menopause is over.

Exercise Is Key for the Mind, Body and Soul

There is no such thing as a healthy lifestyle without exercise. However, the exercise you choose to do has to be enjoyable for you and tweaked in a way that cannot cause you any harm. For instance, if you have a bad back already, you need to alter how you do exercises to avoid putting extra strain on your back and avoid causing any other injuries as a result. If you are not sure how to do this, have a chat with a personal trainer at your gym, or talk to your doctor or physiotherapist. They will be able to give you advice on the best types of exercise for you and how you can modify mainstream exercises to suit your situation and any pre-existing injuries or conditions you have.

It is recommended that adults get around 150 minutes of moderate exercise every week, at least. Alternatively, you can get 75 minutes per week of higher intensity exercise. This type of activity requires you to move your body faster, get your heart rate up and sweat a little. This does not have to be every single day. You can focus on the moderate or the intense exercises or mix them together in a full workout that you do less often. It is up to you how you want to approach your exercise regime.

To make it a long-term plan, you need to fit your workout into your lifestyle and routine. It is better and more beneficial to exercise a little every day, rather than doing a full-on workout once or twice a week. If you spread it out over the week, you are getting continual benefits.

A little later, I will talk about the types of exercise you might like to try and why they are useful for menopausal women, but for now let me give you some idea of what moderate and intense exercise look like.

With moderate exercise, you will be able to talk while you are doing it, but not hold a full conversation. You can say a few words if you need to and will not be out of breath as a result.

Intense exercise means that you need to stop to breathe in between words because it is not possible to speak while you are doing it. These exercise types need to be aerobic, i.e. you are getting your heart rate up and you are sweating a little. It could mean walking fast, jogging, running on the spot, etc. You should also do some form of strengthening exercise ideally twice per week. This will ensure that you are maintaining your muscle mass, which reduces the chances of putting on weight, and strengthening your bones at the same time.

You might be wondering what strengthening exercises look like? The most basic strengthening exercises include push-ups, sit-ups and arm lifts with small hand weights.

It is important to mention that moderate and intense types of exercises are both equally beneficial for menopausal women.

You might be surprised to hear that exercise is not just beneficial for your body, but it is also a fantastic way to keep your spirits up. If you think back to our chapter on stress management, exercise was one of the main ways to keep stress and low mood at bay.

When you exercise, your body releases several feel-good chemicals such as endorphins and dopamine, known to make you feel a natural high. This is partly to help your body to handle the exercise you are doing, but it has the beneficial side effect of boosting your mood at the same time. The more regularly you exercise, the more often you experience this natural high and the better you feel in general.

Of course, low mood and anxiety are common symptoms for menopausal women, so exercising regularly can help you handle these in addition to keeping menopausal weight gain down and strengthening the body.

Be determined to exercise regularly over the next couple of weeks and think honestly about how you feel afterwards. Sure, you might have to wash your sweaty clothes a little more often, but that is a small price to pay when you consider the feel-good factor you will experience as a result!

So, what are the actual benefits of exercise in detail?

Weight Control

It goes without saying that if you eat a healthy diet and exercise regularly, you will likely lose excess weight and keep your weight down. Exercise is a vital weapon in the battle against obesity, but you need to be sure that you are eating healthily alongside it. No amount of exercise will allow you to burn off the calories you consumed if you eat pizza, cakes and burgers every day.

Heart Disease Risk Reduction

The risk of developing heart disease and associated complications are often present as we become a little older, especially as we enter the menopause.

Decreased levels of oestrogen during the menopause can cause LDL cholesterol to rise. That is a "bad type" of cholesterol that is harmful to us and can lead to heart attack and stroke. Exercise plays a vital role in reducing that risk.

When you exercise, you increase the amount of oxygen in your body and improve circulation. Your circulatory system carries oxygen, nutrients and hormones to cells and helps your body to remove carbon dioxide. This plays a part in reducing the risk of heart disease and it also increases the possibility of keeping your body healthy.

Regular exercise can lower your cholesterol and blood pressure. It can also reduce your blood sugar levels, which lowers your risk of becoming obese and developing diabetes. However, this relies upon you eating a healthy diet alongside the exercise.

In addition to these benefits, regular exercise is also believed to reduce your risk of developing certain types of cancer, including breast, uterine, lung and colon cancer.

Mood Improvement and Anxiety Reduction

As I have already mentioned, it is not unusual for a woman to feel down, stressed or anxious during the menopause. It is a result of hormonal changes, the overall stress of what is happening within her body, and could also be from not sleeping well.

Exercise can help you manage this and lift your mood. You will also feel more positive about the changes that are happening inside your body and find it easier to cope with the process as a result.

As I already mentioned, when you exercise, your body releases feel-good chemicals. You will smile more and feel happier, and the effects will last long after you have taken your last movement and sat down for a break. You will feel relaxed and have a sense of achievement too. This all helps you deal with the menopausal symptoms and keep your mood and general feel-good factor up. After endorphins are released inside your body, you will be in a better mood and have more energy as a result. This happy feeling can last for hours after exercising.

Serotonin is another happy hormone that can be affected by exercise. Studies show that cardio exercises are great for boosting serotonin levels, which not only positively affect your mood, but make a difference to your sleep, sexual desire, memory, appetite and digestion.

Mind Strengthening

Brain function is a "use it or lose it" kind of deal and it is essential to regularly challenge yourself to keep your cognitive function up to optimal levels. This applies to any age, but when you are going through the menopause, the hormonal rollercoaster and brain fog you experience make it difficult to concentrate or focus.

When we exercise, the body drives oxygen and blood to the brain, keeping the mind sharper. During exercise, the body releases proteins and endorphins. These not only make us feel good and help strengthen and improve brain function, but they also improve blood circulation, which benefits the brain and improves its sharpness.

Bones and Muscles Strengthening

I have mentioned that women lose muscle mass during the menopause, leading to possible weight gain and weakening of the bones and developing osteoporosis in later life.

Regular exercise can reduce this risk by keeping your muscles and bones as strong as possible. As a result, your bone density levels will be higher, and your muscle mass will remain optimal, which will help you control weight gain.

Sleep Improvement

While it is not a good idea to exercise right before you sleep (endorphins will flood your body making you feel too active to fall asleep), regular exercise during the day can help you relax and, therefore, sleep better.

Ensuring you get enough exercise throughout the week while checking your sleeping routine (more on that shortly) can allow you to fall asleep much faster than otherwise, avoiding those annoying nights of broken sleep.

All of this means you will be more energised, focused and able to handle the challenges that the menopause may bring. From a weight management point of view, sleep is also vital.

Libido Improvement

Due to the lowered oestrogen and progesterone levels you will experience during menopause, you may find that your desire for sexual intercourse is a lot lower than usual. It might be up and down and all over the place, but you will find that these levels are improved by exercising regularly. This is all down to increased circulation and those feel-good chemicals. Whether this is a plus point for you or not is a personal matter, but it can certainly be a valuable benefit for many.

As you can see, exercise has a range of benefits, not only for the body but for the mind and soul too. You will feel better, be more relaxed, look better, be stronger, and you will be able to manage your weight much more effectively. Again, it is vital that you combine exercise with a healthy diet – one does not work without the other, so make sure that you are ticking both boxes to receive the significant benefits on offer.

Exercise is one thing you can do for free that will make many of your menopausal symptoms more manageable.

As you will see in the next sections, you can add extra enjoyment to it by working with a friend or merely finding an activity that interests you.

Finding Your Perfect Exercise

There are countless types of exercise you can try, and you can stick to the kind of exercise you like, or you can mix things up occasionally. You do not need to do anything you do not enjoy, so if you are not a fan of going to the gym, you do not have to go. If you are not a fan of getting into a swimsuit, no-one is forcing you to. If you want, you can download an app on your smartphone and try yoga in the comfort of your home. There are no rules to this; you simply go with what feels right to you.

There is a myth that exercising has to be hard work, you have to sweat, wear rather unflattering lycra, and spend a small fortune on a gym membership, which you must use several times per week without fail. None of this is true.

Yes, exercise is hard work, but it can be done in a way that makes it feel less so, by doing something you enjoy. Nobody is pushing you to join a gym if you are not keen or if you simply cannot afford the rather costly membership fees.

If you would rather exercise in the comfort of your own home than in public, I recommend you read my book, *Get Fit and Healthy in Your Own Home in 20 Minutes or Less*. In this book, you will find a daily exercise plan with plenty of home workouts and simple meal ideas to help you lose weight and get the body you want. The exercises I shared in this book are easy to follow and suitable for the needs of menopausal women. The book is available on Amazon.

Living healthily does not need to be expensive or time consuming, but one thing that a healthy lifestyle needs from you is your commitment. You need to commit to eating nutritious foods and moving your body as often as you can. You must also remember to include other aspects of self-care. They are equally important.

There are countless ways you can weave exercise into your routine and many small things you can do every day to get your body moving more. These are the types of things we will talk about in this section.

The bottom line is that even small changes to your daily routine can make a difference. Here are a few suggestions:

- Walk to work rather than use the car.

- Get off the bus a couple of stops earlier than you usually would and walk the rest of the way.

- Take the steps instead of the lift.

- Go for a walk on your lunch break, rather than sit at your desk.

- When you talk to friends on the phone, walk around the room as you do it, rather than sit on the sofa.

- Washing your car is another excellent way of getting a full-body exercise that works with most of your muscle groups, particularly your upper body: chest, shoulders and arms.

- Gardening is another great way of implementing movement in your everyday life.

I have just shown you that even if you never place a foot inside the gym, there are many things you can do to keep your body in shape.

Of course, we know that it is important you also have to do some formal exercise, i.e. an activity which gets your blood flowing and your heart rate up. While going through the menopause, many women feel unsure of their health because so many changes are occurring at the same time. Doing regular exercise can help any person improve their health, and it is very common for the exercise to alleviate some of the symptoms associated with the menopause. Trust me on this!

In this book, I am not promoting any specific activity, as it is up to you which one you go for, but the following are a few suggestions which may be useful for menopausal women in particular.

I would like to remind you that before you start with any type of exercise, it is important to have a quick chat with your doctor if you have any pre-existing conditions or any specific limitations in your mobility, e.g. a regularly sore back or arthritis.

Doing exercises that are not suitable for your condition could be quite damaging. Make sure that you always look after your body.

- *Join an exercise class* – By joining a class, you gain an extra boost in confidence because it is a social activity at the same time. If you opt for a class for your particular age group, you will probably feel more comfortable. How about Zumba or even belly dancing? Go for something you have always wanted to try but never felt able to and see how great it feels when you master a new activity.

- **_Brisk walking outdoors_** – Heading outdoors means you are getting a boost of vitamin D and serotonin from the sun, but always remember to practice sun safety. Brisk walking is also a great way to get some aerobic exercise, working your lungs and getting your heart rate up. This helps to burn calories and therefore manage your weight. Of course, aerobic exercise also helps to protect against heart disease. If you want to add a touch of strength training, you simply need to carry a small set of hand weights as you are walking.

- **_Hiking_** – If you love the outdoors and you are relatively fit, why not put on your walking boots and head out into the countryside, to the coast, or the nearest mountain? This is a great way to get all the benefits of being outside while enjoying aerobic exercise. Of course, be sure to check the weather and always listen to your body.

- **_Jogging_** – If you have never tried jogging before, start slow and build up as you go. Head to the nearest park and enjoy the scenery while grabbing some much-needed aerobic exercise. This can also help build up strength in the legs, contributing to muscle and bone health. It is perfectly fine to do spurts of just 10 minutes, which should be achievable after a few introductory sessions if you have never done jogging before. All you need to do is do three sets and rest between intervals to take you up to your half an hour of aerobic exercise a day.

- **Swimming** – Swimming is the ideal combination of strength training and aerobic exercise because of the water-resistance. We know that strength training is vital for menopausal women to prevent bone density loss and preserves as much muscle mass as possible. Swimming is probably one of the most gentle ways to achieve this type of exercise. Of course, being in the water is also very calming and relaxing, which could help you deal with any anxiety you may be experiencing and help you get a good night's sleep.

- **Join the gym** – If you want to try joining the gym, then go for it. Most gyms have introductory sessions and you have the services of a personal trainer or instructor to hand if you want further advice. This can be useful if you have never really used gym equipment before and if you have any conditions that mean specific exercises need to be adapted for your needs. You also get the option of using machinery to help with strength training while combining it with your aerobic needs.

- **Yoga and Pilates** – Yoga and Pilates are both ideal activities for menopausal women because they help with flexibility and strength while also building muscle mass. Of course, they are both very relaxing activities, especially yoga, which teaches you to focus on breathing to overcome difficulties and help you move into various positions. There is a suggestion that yoga can help with sleep issues by relaxing you and easing sore muscles that may be holding tension. If you have any problems with mobility, it is crucial to speak to the instructor before the class begins, and they will show you how to alter the poses for your particular needs.

- **Join the club** – Joining your local tennis or golf club is a great idea. There are many sports you can start playing at any age. I named two of them as an example, but nothing stops you from joining any club and starting a new sport. It does not matter if your age is 40-plus or 50-plus; learning a sport you have never played before will raise your confidence and help you develop new skills. It will also build your fitness level, improve your health and maintain a healthy weight. Of course, you also get to meet new people there.

This is not an exhaustive list of sporting activities you can try, but those mentioned are specifically useful for women of a menopausal age because they help to reduce many menopausal symptoms and offer a combination of aerobic and strength exercises.

Do not Overdo It!

There is a common way of thinking that you need to be "all in" when it comes to exercise, but that is not the case. As long as you are doing as much as you can do comfortably and you are doing it regularly, that is enough. You do not have to push yourself to extremes. You are only going to end up injured or develop aches and pains if you do.

It is vital that before you start any exercise session, regardless of what it is, you do some stretches to warm your muscles up. If you go into your exercise cold, you might end up with a pulled muscle and possibly worse. Your body is already under enough stress at this time of your life, so do not add extra fuel to the fire by attempting to exercise without warming up. Warm-up exercises are designed to warm your muscles and prepare your body for exercise. Stretches are easy enough to do and you should not overextend to the point of pain either — simply feeling a gentle pull is all you need.

You should also stretch after you have exercised; this is called a cool down. Stretching exercises relax and restore your muscles after the workout. This helps your muscles remain flexible, which can be a problem during menopause. If you do not do this, your muscles will feel tight and painful the next day, and perhaps you will struggle to move.

Cooling down helps protect the wide range of motion in all major muscle groups and ensures that your joints remain flexible and healthy. Remember, these are areas of the body that can deteriorate as you age. While I am not suggesting that you are ready to start drawing your pension payments, you do need to start protecting your body for your later years — the ideal time is now.

Stretching also helps with stability, which will help you when you get much older and may be more susceptible to falls. Being flexible and supple is never a bad thing, and you will feel fitter and healthier for far longer by following this advice.

In the book I mentioned earlier, *Get Fit and Healthy in Your Own Home in 20 Minutes or Less*, you will find plenty of warm-up and stretching exercises. Both types of exercises can prevent your body from strain and injuries and keep it in good form.

It goes without saying that you should stay hydrated during your exercise sessions and make sure that you drink plenty of water. If you feel lightheaded or you are sweating excessively, sit down and take a break. You should not feel this way during regular exercise.

Do not push yourself to your extreme limits; you simply need to move your body more and get your heart rate up a little. That is all! Anything more than that and you are putting yourself at risk of injury and illness — and that is not what we are aiming for.

Remember, your body is under enough stress as it is; you simply need to take some of the strain away by helping it out with some healthy exercise along with a healthy diet. By trying to do too much, especially if you have never really had an exercise routine before, you are going to end up feeling terrible afterwards and probably be put off exercising ever again.

Moving your body and exercising regularly is the key to your success — remember this! Overdoing it once in a while or pushing yourself to the extreme levels on a daily basis is not what your body needs. The key is to find an exercise that you enjoy, dedicate time to it and make it a priority. If exercising feels like a chore and you are dreading exercise time or simply do not enjoy what you are doing, you have likely chosen the wrong type of exercise. I suggest you think again and look at different options.

Exercising is something you need to feel happy and comfortable doing over the long term. Doing the right type of exercise is crucial. When you do something you love, you will feel happier and more positive. Feeling this way will motivate you to create a habit of exercising regularly.

Finding an Exercise Buddy

Many women find exercising alone to be a lonely business. Of course, not everyone feels this way, but if you do, why not find an exercise buddy and make your active time a social time too? This can be ideal for banishing stress, and if you exercise with another woman your age, you can share your experiences of the menopause with each other. You will be able to understand each other's struggles.

Exercising with other people is the reason why many women choose to attend an exercise class. If you look around your local area, I am sure you will find classes catering only for women over the age of 40 or 50. This could help you meet other women who are going through this time in life and give you support. Besides, other people can motivate us when we are feeling tired, uninspired or lazy.

Making exercise fun is not as difficult as you think. Yes, your muscles might burn and you are going to be a little out of breath, but as I mentioned before, if you choose an exercise that you enjoy, you will not notice the downsides. You are also strengthening your body and helping to maintain your weight. That pesky menopausal weight gain issue is something which most women deal with, but exercise, along with a healthy diet, will help you to master the problem with far greater ease than otherwise.

So, how else can you make exercise fun?

- **Download a tracking app** – Many women like to use pedometers, but how about downloading an app that measures how many steps you are taking throughout the day. There are apps that could help you compete against family or friends, measuring who makes a higher number of steps per day. That is a great motivator and an excellent way to make exercise fun and competitive, rather than something you simply have to do.

- **Make sure you go outside** – Again, we have talked about this, but it is vital to put it in this section too. Exercising outdoors makes it more fun because of the fresh air and the new environment, and it is excellent for your mood. Natural light and fresh air can boost your immune system and strengthen your mental health, which will benefit you while navigating the menopausal journey.

- **Exercise at different times of the day** – Mix your routine up and exercise at different times. Doing this can stop your exercise routine from becoming tedious and help you discover your favourite time of the day to exercise. You might be doing it in the morning simply because you think that is the best time, but if you do not try a few different options, how will you really know? When you find your favourite time to exercise, then stick to it and put it in your diary.

- **Keep an exercise journal** – When you choose a new exercise or activity, it is a good idea to keep a journal and write down your experiences. Journaling will help you understand how you feel about it and whether it is the right one for you.

Should you weigh yourself every day?

I do not recommend you weigh yourself too often. Our weight fluctuates naturally throughout the day and even across the week, so weighing yourself every day is going to give you unhelpful information. If you do not see the results you want, it could damage your confidence.

Weigh yourself once a week and always do it at the same time, simply so you know whether your weight is going up, down, or it is staying the same. Whatever the number you see on the scale, do not allow it to upset you. Weight loss is a journey like any other — sometimes smooth and sometimes rough. The changes you are going to make to your lifestyle will be far-reaching, and that is something you need to have faith in at this point.

Weighing yourself daily could be disempowering if you do not see a massive difference in numbers, but do not panic; it is better to measure your progress according to how you feel. This is the advice I always give to my clients.

Instead of focusing on the number on the scale, I suggest you pay attention to the following:

- Do you have more energy?

- Are you sleeping better?

- What are your menopausal symptoms like at this point?

The weight loss will come as you continue with your healthy lifestyle via a balanced diet and regular exercise. When you are preparing healthy foods or sweating on the gym floor or in the park, think about all the health benefits you are achieving by doing this, rather than how much you weigh.

The way we feel is much more important. Besides, fat loss sometimes comes before weight loss. This means that your clothes will fit you better, your posture will improve, but the scale will show the opposite. This is the harsh reality of weight loss. That is why you should not focus solely on the number on the scale but also on the positive side effects of your healthy lifestyle and healthy attitude towards your body.

I previously mentioned an exercise journal and also talked about a food journal that could help you find out how different foods make you feel. You can combine these journals to look at patterns and spot trends.

When you do weigh yourself, jot these numbers down and look for the downward trend. If you notice the numbers going up a little, you can search through your journal for any clues as to why this is the case.

Some of my clients tell me that they are finding it more challenging to lose weight, and sometimes they even notice their weight went up following a period of poor sleep.

The lack of sleep contributes to their low energy levels, so they exercise less. Poor sleep is also associated with consuming more sugary loaded foods and simple carbohydrates. Unhealthy food choices are often linked to increased levels of ghrelins — a hunger hormone caused by a lack of sleep.

I already talked about the importance of good sleep, and I highly recommend focusing on it as a main priority. Without proper rest, you might find it very hard to have a healthy body and a healthy mind. We will talk more about this topic in the next chapter.

Remember, you are aiming for a new lifestyle for the rest of your years, not for just a few weeks or months.

Key Points

In this chapter, I have talked at length about exercise. You might not have initially loved the idea of being more active, but I hope I have inspired you to think about taking up a new activity or perhaps re-starting one which you may have done in the past.

I want you to remember these key points from this section:

- Exercise is vital for overall health and well-being and is an essential tool in managing your weight.

- Regular exercise has a range of benefits, including weight management, reducing the risk of heart disease, promoting better sleep and strengthening bones and muscles. All of these benefits are vital for a menopausal woman.

- It is no good exercising if you are not eating in the right way. Regular exercise and healthy eating need to be close partners if you want to gain the greatest benefits.

- Find an exercise activity that you enjoy — exercise should not be a chore; it should be something you like to do and something which makes you feel good.

- Remember to have a combination of aerobic and strength training exercises and always warm up and cool down too.

- If you are starting a new exercise activity and have a condition or pre-existing injury, consult your doctor to find out how you can adapt the exercise to suit your needs.

Chapter 6

Sleep Your Way to Weight Loss?

Who does not love a good night's sleep?

That wonderful feeling when you wake up in the morning, look at your alarm clock and realise that you have another three hours before you have to get up. Ahh, bliss! You turn back over, snuggling into your duvet and allow yourself to drift back off.

Sleep is not just an enjoyable thing; it is also vital for having a healthy body and mind. We need sleep for a very good reason. Unfortunately, during the menopause, many women find their sleep pattern disturbed and some may even struggle with insomnia.

Why is this?

Again, it is attributed to hormones and how they affect the human body. I have already mentioned that as you enter the menopause, the two primary hormones, progesterone and oestrogen, start to dwindle. The problem is, progesterone is the hormone that helps you fall asleep. So, when it is in low supply, you begin to struggle with getting a good night's sleep. You might find it hard to fall asleep, or wake up several times during the night, thereby leaving you feeling exhausted the next day.

Night sweats can also be a problem when you are trying to sleep. When this happens, your body is experiencing a quick hit of adrenaline, and again, that is not conducive to relaxation and sleep. It is part and parcel of the fight or flight stress response I talked about earlier. Experiencing night sweats several times per night and over a long period of time (with some women it lasts for months or even years), as we already know, can become dangerous in terms of a prolonged stress response and a lack of sleep.

You might also struggle with sleep as a result of anxiety. It is normal to feel worried and confused during any changes in your life, and the menopause is a pretty big one. In this case, you may find yourself overthinking when you are at your quietest moment, meaning that you struggle to go to sleep or have difficult dreams.

Of course, it is crucial that you do your best to have as good a night's sleep as possible. We all need to rest. During sleep, the body focuses on regeneration, healing, and replenishing energy for the next day. In addition, your body is changing, which means you need to rest to allow it to complete the process it needs to go through.

In this chapter, I am going to talk in more detail about how you can make changes in your lifestyle to help you find the sweet spot for sleep.

The Undeniable Connection Between Sleep and Weight

Sleep, sleep, sleep... It is essential not only for managing your weight loss but also for maintaining your overall health and well-being. Many health conditions can be improved simply by getting better rest on a more consistent basis. If you are not sleeping well, your immune system will be affected, and you will be more at risk of developing some life-threatening conditions. Also, you are more likely to put weight on. Have you noticed this?

Sleep was one of the few things that our parents made sure we had enough of when we were babies, but we all tend to abandon it when we reach our teenage years. This is quite possibly one of the first good habits we give up on in life.

Establishing a consistent sleep schedule will help you get a better sleep quality every night, helping you be the best version of yourself each day.

One of the best analogies I have ever heard compared sporadic bedtimes to jet lag. Whether you lose 3 hours or 13 hours to a flight, you know your entire body simply feels off when you jump through time zones. Every time you go to sleep one hour later than usual, your natural rhythm is disrupted.

We have become so used to feeling like this that now we assume it is perfectly normal. In fact, sleeping more hours and having a better quality of sleep will provide us with better health and more energy.

Numerous studies show the positive effects of sleep on our well-being and many found a strong correlation between lack of sleep and weight gain.

In 2013, a study conducted by the University of Colorado investigated how sleep affects eating and gaining weight. The results concluded that sleeping just five hours a night over only one week leads to putting on around two pounds in weight. According to these findings, it would mean that if you sleep that long every night over a month, that is eight pounds in weight, gained simply by not sleeping enough.

The study showed that your hunger signals simply do not shut off when you do not get enough sleep, leading you to consume extra 500-plus calories in one day.

The average adult is supposed to get between seven to eight hours of sleep every night. Of course, most people do not hit that spot every night, but on average, that is the best duration we should aim for. Anything less than that will have an impact on our health, energy, or mood.

The problem of weight gain comes when there is a lack of sleep, i.e. you are sleep deprived. You are classed as being sleep deprived when you get less sleep than the seven to eight hours recommended, even for just a few nights, and you are experiencing the following symptoms:

- Feeling very sleepy during the daytime

- Excessive yawning

- Feeling moody or snappy

- Forgetting things easily

- General fatigue

- Low mood

- Not being able to concentrate or handle anything new which is presented to you, i.e. difficulty taking on new ideas or concepts

Some of those symptoms overlap with the menopause, making it challenging to figure out the real problem. However, if you are finding it hard to fall asleep, you wake up often, you do not want to get out of bed in the mornings and you are struggling with tiredness throughout the day, I advise you to change your routine and do your best to address your sleep problem.

When you are sleep deprived, some hormonal imbalances occur within your body. I am talking here about hunger and satiation hormones, ghrelin and leptin. When you are not getting enough sleep, the levels of these two hormones are affected. Therefore, you feel hungrier, and your body does not notice when you are full quite as easily.

Here is a brief explanation of how they work and how they are affected by your sleep.

Ghrelin is the hormone that is responsible for telling your brain when you need to eat. And leptin tells your brain when you are full. In other words, ghrelin increases the appetite, while leptin decreases the appetite.

During a good night's sleep, the ghrelin levels will decrease, and leptin levels will increase. If you did not have a good night's sleep, your hormones would be affected, and your ghrelin levels will be increased, which means that you will be eating more. On the other hand, your leptin levels will be decreased. Therefore, your body will not know when it is full, and as a result, you will feel hungrier and eat more before feeling full up.

This is the perfect storm for weight gain because it leads you to make unhealthy food choices and overeat. As I have mentioned before, you are more likely to be tempted towards foods which are high in unhealthy fat and sugar and of course, these are the types of foods that will make you pile on the pounds. The fact that you are sleep deprived means that you cannot make clear and sensible decisions, so you are more likely to overeat too. Many studies have shown this, and unfortunately, I experienced it myself.

We also know that getting older affects your muscle mass, and from the age of 30 we begin to lose muscle mass by 3-8% per decade. After the age of 60, the rate we lose muscle mass is increased. But do not worry! It has been proven that leading a healthy lifestyle can help us build muscle at any age. Including good nutrition and regular exercise in your daily routine you can reverse the process and slow down muscle mass decrease.

Sleep is another essential factor that is crucial for maintaining muscle mass. When you are not getting enough sleep, the muscle mass is at a critical level. The lower your muscle mass, the more difficult it will be to maintain your healthy weight.

As you can see, sleep is vital and not just something we like to do at night when we are feeling a little tired and want to forget about the day's worries. The good news is that if you are having problems with sleep during your menopausal period, there are many things you can do to change your lifestyle and give yourself a better chance of having a full seven to eight hours of sleep every night.

10 Ways to Get a Better Night's Sleep

In this section, I am going to talk to you about changing your routine to increase your chances of getting a good night's sleep regularly. You might not struggle with sleep every night, but most women going through the menopause have disturbances at some point, either every few nights or for a prolonged period.

Establishing a routine prepares the body and brain for falling asleep faster; therefore, I suggest you explore the ideas I am going to share with you. These methods are worth looking into even if some of the problems I mentioned do not apply to you.

Go to Bed and Wake up At the Same Time Every Day

You might be tempted to have a lie-in at the weekend, but I would not suggest it. It is a better idea to maintain a routine when it comes to sleep. That means going to bed at the same time every day and setting your alarm for the same time every day too. Sure, it is not going to hurt if you have a special function to attend and go to bed a little later one night, but anything more than that will start sending you into sleep deprivation territory.

Going to bed at the same time, and getting the same amount of sleep every night will make you feel remarkably more alert and energised, and probably help you get slimmer and healthier too. Your body clock is consistent by maintaining a routine, and your hormones will remain in sync far more easily.

Balanced hormones support your physical, mental, and emotional state, and allow you to thrive.

Avoid Anything Too Stimulating Before Bed

It is not a good idea to watch TV till late at night, listen to fast or loud music, or spend hours on your laptop or tablet before you sleep. Instead, listen to chilled out music, read a book and have a warm bath before bedtime. These activities will put you in a more relaxed frame of mind and help you to wind down. Anything too stimulating will just make it harder for you to switch off and will keep you awake.

Rigorous exercising just before bedtime is not advisable. This can raise your cortisol and adrenaline levels. These stress hormones can keep you awake. It is recommended to exercise earlier in the day if at all possible, especially if you have sleeping problems. Exercises that I suggest you do before bedtime are yoga and stretching. Yoga might be able to calm your mind; therefore, it can help you to sleep better. Stretching can relieve muscle tension, which can also help your body to relax.

Try to have at least 30 minutes of quiet time before going to sleep, to let your mind calm down from the day's excitement and entertainment.

Get into the habit of listening to a guided meditation or adult bedtime story before bed to help your nervous system slow down and prepare your brain for sleep.

Ideally, have it downloaded to your device so that you can turn off the screen and place it on aeroplane mode.

The more comfortable and relaxed you are before you try to sleep, the better the chances are that you are going to nod off quickly and stay that way until morning.

Avoid Eating Too Close to Bedtime

If your bedtime is 10 p.m., it is a good idea to have dinner no later than 7 p.m. if possible. It is no fun trying to sleep when you are bloated; you are more likely to stay awake, toss, and turn.

I strongly suggest that you avoid eating for at least three hours before going to bed because this gives your body the chance to digest the food and prevents indigestion and stomach-ache.

I also advise you not to drink anything an hour or two before going to bed. One of the most common reasons for disturbed sleep is having to use the toilet in the middle of the night and then not fall back asleep.

Avoid Caffeine and Alcohol

Drinking alcohol later at night is known to disrupt sleep patterns. It has been suggested to stop drinking caffeine at least six hours before you are ready to sleep.

Avoid anything containing caffeine or alcohol and instead opt for a warm, milky drink before you sleep or herbal tea such as chamomile. This will help relax you, making it easier for the dopamine to kick in (a hormone you need at this point), which helps you to sleep.

If you consume alcohol or caffeine:

- You are probably going to be up several times during the night to use the toilet.

- These are stimulants which will simply make you wide awake, rather than fast asleep.

- These can raise your blood sugar levels and negatively impact your sleep and overall health.

Never Take Your Phone to Bed with You

Having your phone underneath your pillow might seem practical, but it is a big distraction, as you are more likely to wake up whenever you hear a beep or feel a vibration.

Turn your phone off or put it on silent and keep it far away from your bed. If you are worried about oversleeping, set an old-fashioned alarm clock!

By having your phone next to you when you are trying to sleep, you are also more likely to start scrolling through social media, which will keep you awake.

Check the Temperature of Your Room

If your room is too hot or too cold, you will not find it easy to sleep properly. Try to adjust your room temperature so that it gets cooler at night, mimicking your body's natural temperature control. This increases melatonin production, which is a sleep hormone that tells your brain it is time to sleep. If the room is too hot or too stuffy, open a window or use a fan; if it is too cold, add some blankets rather than turning up the heating, which will just add to the stuffiness. You could also use an electric blanket, but do not sleep with it turned on all night; simply turn it on for an hour before you are going to sleep and then you will be warm and toasty.

Check Your Sleeping Environment

Aside from the temperature, check your bed and how comfortable it is. Does the mattress need turning? Do you need extra or fewer blankets? Is there something about the material of the blankets that bothers you? Are you allergic to feathers in the pillows?

Make sure your mattress is appropriate for your unique sleeping needs. Investing in a mattress that works for you can improve your sleep quality, so it is worth considering it. You should also check how long you have had your pillows for, as these do need to be changed regularly if you want them to be comfortable and supportive. A year or two is the maximum you should keep these.

Try a Weighted Blanket

Weighted blankets are regularly used to treat restless legs syndrome (RLS), but they are also useful for anyone who simply struggles with sleep.

In this case, the blanket is heavier, and you can choose which weight you want it to be. The idea is that the blanket is like a hug, and as a result your body releases oxytocin, which is another hormone naturally occurring within the body. This hormone helps you relax and feel content, which is ideal for helping you get to sleep.

Keep a Pen and Paper Beside Your Bed

A good idea is to keep a pen and paper beside your bed. If you wake up with something you do not want to forget, scribble it down and work on it the next day. By simply writing it down, you have cast it from your mind and you will feel freer as a result. There is nothing more distracting when you are trying to sleep than remembering something and then feeling worried that you are going to forget it.

I find this tip very useful. As a writer, I always have lots of ideas going through my head. Not writing them down would prevent me from sleeping. Therefore, this works for me.

Try Lavender Oil

It goes without saying that you should check with your doctor if you have any problems, allergies, or taking any medications before trying any holistic or alternative therapies. If you are good to go, a lavender essential oil is a great go-to.

You could add a few drops to a warm bath before bed, try a pillow mist, or simply add a few drops to a tissue and leave it beside your pillow. Some people also find it useful to add a drop to the soles of their feet or their inner wrists, but in this case, you should water the oil down with a carrier oil, as undiluted essential oil can be damaging to the skin.

Lavender oil is known to relax and induce sleep while also being fantastic for anxiety and stress. Scents such as lavender, chamomile and sage have also been shown to have calming aromatic properties.

Sleep can help your body in so many ways. During this time, the body restores and rebalances itself. To achieve a good quality sleep it is vital to create the right environment, so your body can relax and you can have a good night's sleep. The number of hours you need to sleep every night depends on your individual needs.

Is Insomnia a Real Problem for You?

You might be confused about the difference between sleep deprivation and insomnia. The lines are quite blurred, but if you are struggling with sleep and nothing is making it better, you should certainly visit your doctor and discuss therapies or treatments which may improve your situation. Sleep deprivation over a long period, i.e. insomnia, is not something you should have to deal with.

If you are struggling with insomnia you will need to speak to your doctor about it. They will ask you a series of questions and perhaps even offer sleep studies to determine the cause. However, this is more likely to happen if the problem is exceptionally prolonged or if you are suffering from other sleep-related issues, such as sleep apnea.

The bottom line is that if you are struggling with sleep, you need to make some lifestyle changes first and foremost and see if that makes a difference.

Many menopausal women find that their sleep is disturbed on and off throughout this time. It is not usually an ongoing and prolonged issue that drastically reduces your sleep, but if you are struggling and your life is affected by the lack of sleep, you need to get extra help to sort the problem out.

You might think that sleep is not important and that you are wasting your doctor's time, but you are not. Having a good night's sleep is crucial for many reasons. During this time your body gets a break from digesting the food and coping with stress. Remember that your body is the machine that never stops working. Sleep offers your body a chance to tidy up and restore, which reduces inflammation and supports healing.

Sleep is a vital part of your life, and it is something that your brain and body need in order to stay fit and healthy. Of course, there is the weight gain side of the coin to consider too. Gaining weight due to the lack of sleep and subsequent unhealthy food choices means that you are also putting your health at risk. For all of these reasons, you need to make sleep a priority and work out how to make your situation better.

Key Points

In this chapter, I have talked about sleep and why the menopause may affect it. And we looked at the link between sleep and weight gain. The good news is that you can reverse this link by making some changes to your lifestyle, which will help you rectify your sleep problem.

The main points to remember from this chapter are:

- Sleep can be disturbed during the menopause.

- Sleep deprivation affects the levels of leptin and ghrelin within the body, which means that you are more likely to put on weight through unhealthy food choices.

- Hot flushes and night sweats can affect sleep, so you should try and remain as cool as possible and avoid hot drinks. Monitor the temperature of your room, and if necessary open the window.

- If you are struggling with insomnia, i.e. you are not sleeping well and are always tired during the day, you should see your doctor and find out what can help solve your problem.

- Most sleep problems can be solved or improved with a few changes to your lifestyle.

- Avoid overstimulating yourself before you sleep and look towards relaxation instead.

- You must go to bed and wake up at the same time every day, to ensure that your body clock remains regular and your hormones are therefore regulated far more easily.

- Progesterone is naturally lower during the menopause, and this is a hormone which is related to sleep.

- Sleep is a vital function for the brain and body, so never feel awkward or embarrassed to talk about it. During this time, your brain and your body are healing, regenerating, and getting ready for the next day. It is impossible to function effectively without sleep.

Chapter 7

Finding Support Around You

We are almost at the end of the book. I hope that you are feeling more hopeful and positive about the process that you are currently going through or anticipating. Because that is all it is: a process. Every process eventually comes to an end. Life continues either the same as before or enriched by the experience you have been through.

I sincerely hope that you will find the strength to deal with any difficulties that the menopause causes for you, and learn to see this time in your life as a transition, rather than a definition. I also hope the content in this book has helped you to realise that you can take control of your health, your weight, and your happiness, simply by choosing to take the right kind of action.

In this final chapter, I want to leave you feeling upbeat and positive. I want to give you a last inspiring talk to stay with you long after reading the final words, and I want to recap on the most important points you have learnt.

You do not have to go through the menopause alone. Some women do not want to share this deeply personal time in their life with others and that is perfectly fine, but some women would certainly benefit from talking a little more, sharing stories and perhaps learning coping mechanisms from other menopausal women.

My advice is to look to those around you for support if you feel you need it and travel through the menopause in a way which you think is best for you. There is no right or wrong answer. Go with what feels right.

The Menopause is Neither a Full Stop Nor a Definition

For some women, the most challenging part of the menopause is not the possible weight gain or the possible symptoms you might encounter, but what it stands for. The menopause is, as I have already outlined earlier in the book, the point at which you are no longer fertile; your menstrual cycle ends, and you move on to the next chapter of your life. In its very essence, that chapter does mean that you are moving into the second part of your life. And that is something that many women struggle to come to terms with.

It is all right to feel that way and you are certainly not alone. You need to realise that just because your menstrual cycle has finished and you are no longer releasing eggs to become pregnant, that does not make you any less of a woman. It simply means that your body is going through a cycle.

In many ways, the menopause makes you more of a woman than before, because you have earned your stripes. You have been there; you have done it. You have been through around 40 or so years of having periods every month. You have struggled with finding the right type of contraception and probably dealt with its side effects. You have battled with your hormones and won. You might have had children or maybe you did not, either way, it means that you have lived your fertile years as a woman. And you know what? You deserve to rest now. You deserve not to have to deal with a period every month, powerful contraceptive pills, menstrual cramps and the worry of pregnancy.

While the menopause can be difficult while you are going through it, and it can be a little up and down in the immediate years afterwards, everything will settle down, and you will feel better. This point in your life is not a full stop. It is not the end of anything; it simply means that your ovaries are not releasing eggs, but that should not have a significant impact on your daily life at this point. It is probably unlikely you will be thinking about having children at 50 anyway.

The menopause does not end anything and does not define your womanhood either. The other things in your life define you — your personality, confidence, passion, courage, intuition, kindness, the way you treat other people, the things you are good at, and the mark you leave on the world. Those are more important things to focus on than whether or not you are menstruating every month.

However, I can appreciate that the menopause can change the way a woman sees herself, especially when it comes to menopausal weight gain and how that affects confidence.

Any type of weight gain can be detrimental to confidence levels and when you are feeling low and not too great within yourself, it affects every single aspect of your life. You might start to notice a drop in your mood or become agitated with those around you or avoid social events because you worry about judgement on how you look. You might miss a great opportunity because you do not feel able to complete whatever it is you need to do.

We are always told that beauty is on the inside, and I agree entirely, but there is a lot of truth in the idea that how you feel about yourself is intrinsically tied to your outer appearance too.

My advice is this — make sure you follow the guidance in this book and focus on overall health and well-being. When you do that you really cannot go wrong in any way, you will be healthier, you will feel more energetic, you will be more upbeat, you will have more energy and your confidence levels will soar. Perhaps most pertinently, you will not gain weight because you have regained control over your body and those pesky hormones which create all sorts of problems during this time of your life.

It can be hard to resist temptation when your leptin and ghrelin hormones are totally out of sync, and you are hungry for seemingly no reason. But if you are following a healthy lifestyle, you will be stronger in your mind and feel less inclined to make poor food choices. Instead, you will reach for a snack that will not cause you to gain weight, grab a glass of water to fill you up, or go out for a walk to get some fresh air and therefore overcome the craving without any dietary damage.

The menopause is as much about how you approach it mentally as it is about how you deal with the symptoms on a physical level.

Of course, there is a very emotional side to the menopause too, which also needs addressing.

I want you to understand that the cycle you are going through now is simply part of life and not all of your life. You are not defined or judged on how you dealt with the menopause; nobody is going to talk about how difficult or otherwise you found the change. It is a personal deal that nobody else needs to be a part of unless you want them to be. However, as I will now further elaborate, seeking out support and sharing your feelings is a positive step to take.

Finding Support

As women, we can sometimes have a habit of knocking each other down, but in our more exceptional moments, we can also build each other up. If you reach out to someone to talk and admit that perhaps you are struggling and you need a little help, the chances are that they will be more than willing to lend you an ear, give you some advice and share their experiences. All you need to do is ask.

Some women do sail their way through the menopause without much stress or trouble, but those are in the minority. Many women struggle in some way, and the area in which you struggle is a personal thing.

Some women find that their biggest problem is a lack of sleep, while others cannot control their hunger, and that is massively contributing to their weight gain. Some cannot handle the hot flushes or night sweats, while others find the emotional side of the menopause more troublesome.

Tension or anxiety are common feelings experienced by many women when they reach the menopause. Whatever you are struggling with, I urge you to talk about it and be open about your experiences. By doing that, you are not only helping yourself, but you might also inspire other women who may be struggling and do not have the confidence within themselves to speak up and ask for help.

We live in a world of technology and while social media may be a double-edged sword in many ways, it does have its advantages. One of those aspects is the availability of support groups. Before the days of Facebook, we did not connect with those further away from us very easily. I am not suggesting that we have a smoother ride than women 30 or 40 years ago, but we do have a range of available resources that were unheard of in the past. We can use these resources and the availability of information to our benefit.

Search for Facebook support groups and be brave enough to discuss with other women the ways your body behaves and how you feel about those changes. In these groups, you will meet other like-minded women going through the same thing as you, and you never know, you might meet a new lifelong friend.

These groups do not need to be all doom and gloom. You do not need to share your scare stories of hot flushes and night sweats, but you can talk about any aspects of the menopause you are struggling with and simply work through your issues with people who understand. You will find out about various ways to handle troublesome symptoms from other women in the group and probably feel better knowing that you have others by your side who support you.

You could also talk to your doctor and find out if the surgery is running any support groups, or whether they know of any community-based groups related to women's health. Most regional areas have such groups, and on the whole, you are unlikely to need to travel too far to find one.

If meeting strangers in this way is not for you, that is fine. You do not have to do this if you do not feel comfortable with it. In this case, make sure that you make time for friends and focus on your social life. By doing this, you are taking your mind off the troubles you might be going through, increasing your confidence in the process.

Spending time with friends, laughing, having shared experiences and simply being in the presence of those we enjoy spending time with can be therapy in itself.

You can suggest some of the healthy lifestyle tips I mentioned throughout the book, like going to an exercise class together or perhaps just taking the dogs for a walk and having a chat as you do so.

A big part of dealing with the menopause healthily, avoiding weight gain and feeling confident within yourself is handling the emotional and mental aspects of the process.

The Power of Talking

It is good to talk, right? We are told to talk about how we feel because offloading emotions and problems can help put them into perspective, and the phrase "A problem shared is a problem halved" is true. In this case, you can talk to someone about how you are feeling, without judgement, and you will probably feel 10 times better afterwards. They do not even need to reply in some cases, simply saying the words out loud can be enough.

However, what do you do if you do not want to verbalise how you are feeling to another person?

In that case, start writing a journal. I mentioned journaling a little earlier when talking about food and exercise, but this is a different type of journal. Previously, I spoke about making a record to look for patterns, but the kind of journaling that I am referring to now is a way of getting your feelings out and feeling better for it. You do not have to show anyone this journal. It can be for your eyes only, but if you want to explain to someone how you feel but struggling to find the right words, you could simply pour your heart out on a piece of paper and give it to them instead.

You see, writing is cathartic. It is a way of looking through your feelings and making sense of what is going on inside your mind and within your heart. For the most part, simply writing down your thoughts and feelings can be enough of a release to help you handle the problem more healthily from that point onwards. However, if you feel like you would like another person's input, you simply need to find a person you trust — someone who understands.

There are many worries and concerns which may go through the mind of a menopausal woman. Some women might worry about changes in their appearance and feel concerned about their weight gain or the sudden appearance of wrinkles on their faces due to the low level of oestrogen.

Other women feel emotional and confused about their menopausal symptoms — hot flushes, brain fog, anxiety, thinning hair and dry skin. You might feel anxious about what is going on inside you and wonder why you do not feel *yourself* anymore. If you allow all of this to bottle up, you will become stressed and risk damaging your mental health. It is vital that you talk things through, whether you believe what you are saying is important or not. If it is bothering you, it is important. It is that simple.

Of course, during the menopause, it is not unusual for a woman to experience mood swings and to become agitated for no reason and perhaps to snap or shout at their nearest and dearest. You can blame your hormones for this, but your family and friends might not realise it and could take it quite personally. These outbursts result from the maelstrom of emotions and feelings you are experiencing because your hormones are dictating your every move at this point. But during your calmer moments — and you will have many of these — I suggest you sit down with your loved ones and talk about what is going on and how you feel.

By doing this, they will understand better.

They will perhaps make some concessions for any further outbursts in the future, learn how not to take it personally and not become hurt by you snapping at them for no reason, and you will feel more supported as a result. In this case, the menopause could bring you closer to those around you, but it hinges on your ability to talk about it first and foremost. This is not a taboo subject; it happens to every woman on the planet — nobody gets to escape it.

The menopause is a normal part of life and we should feel able to talk about what is going on and how we feel about the symptoms we experience, without worries over judgement or embarrassment.

Do not block out the people around you. Embrace their support and let them in. They are probably wondering what is going on with you, worrying why you are acting a little differently, or why you seem distracted or down. Talk about it, let them in, allow them to help. Even if they cannot practically help you and take it all away from you, simply talking about it candidly will help you and indirectly, help them.

The Menopause Does Not Last Forever

If there is one message I want to give you at this point, it is the reassurance that this is just a phase in your life and that the menopause does not and is not going to last forever. Sure, when you are lying awake at night suffering from a night sweat, you are probably wondering whether it is ever going to end. When you notice that your trousers are becoming a little tighter and it starts to make you question your appearance, you will wonder what happens and what is about to happen, but remember this — you have control.

The menopause will end, and your symptoms will eventually subside and leave you feeling normal again, whatever that may be. You will also feel yourself once more and are going to have the same — if not better — outlook on life.

I know, it does not seem that way at the moment. You are stressed, tired, confused and probably hungry, but if you follow the advice I have talked you through, you will find your menopausal experience to be far more positive and even uplifting than you could have imagined, before you picked up this book. Once it is all over, you will be healthier as a result.

Remember, the menopause does not last forever; this is just a small part of your life that you are living right now.

The postmenopausal stage has its challenges, but menopausal symptoms will gradually disappear. You can be healthy and feel good about your body despite your biological age. Your health and the quality of life in your later years will depend on the way you live right now. If you focus on self-care, eating healthily and living a healthy lifestyle, you will have a higher chance of enjoying your midlife and beyond.

Take Control of Your Health and Control Your Life

Finally, I want to mention that you have control here. It might seem like your hormones are in control, and to a certain degree they are, but those reins can be totally in your hands if you make the right choices. Choosing how you will live your life and what you are going to eat, how often you are going to exercise, who you are going to spend your time with, how much you are going to allow unfortunate circumstances to affect you, is totally in your control. Understanding this and accepting this challenge will bring incredible changes in your life.

You cannot change the fact that your body is changing as we speak. You cannot change the fact that you are moving towards a point in your life when you will not be ovulating or menstruating anymore. You cannot change the fact that you are becoming a little older. However, you can control any potential weight gain and you can control how you feel. You can do a lot to minimise most of your symptoms too. That puts you firmly in the driver's seat to decide how your menopausal journey goes.

Focusing on consuming foods that nourish your body, exercising regularly and finding activities that you love doing, will help you turn the menopause into a positive experience. By doing this, you are taking control of your life and that will feel fantastic. Of course, you do not need to be going through the menopause to do this, but what a great excuse!

Being kind to yourself and taking care of your body is a valuable experience and it is a gift that only you can give to yourself. This experience is something that you can learn a lot from, and you will also learn a lot about yourself and your needs throughout the entire process. Remember, you are in charge and your behavior will determine how well and healthy you are going to be. You cannot rely on other people to take care of your body. You need to take responsibility and do the best you can in order to give yourself a chance to feel well, look good and be proud of yourself.

By acting this way, you are going to be the healthiest you have ever been. Does this idea not make you feel excited? Does it not make you feel eager to get started?

Key Points

I hope that by the end of this chapter, you feel better about the changes you are experiencing in your life right now. Have some faith that this will not be forever and it is simply a stage in your life that you have to go through. Do you remember the time when you got your first period? Can you remember how scary and weird it all felt? Can you remember how everything felt like it was changing for a while afterwards?

Well, in some ways the menopause is a little like that, but the opposite situation. Rather than beginning your fertility journey, it has now come to an end. However, that does not need to be a full stop on your journey as a woman; it is simply a part of your life. The menopause does not have to be any kind of ending, but the beginning of a new life cycle.

Here are the main points to take from this chapter:

- The menopause does not last forever; what you are feeling now will end.

- Finding support from other women going through the same experiences as you can help you boost your confidence and give you a sounding board when you are struggling with a problematic symptom or with general worries and concerns.

- Search online for communities of people to talk to. You can also look for community groups in your local area.

- Meeting other women going or having gone through the menopause will help you build up your confidence and give your life a social boost.

- Do not shut out your family and friends. They may be worried about why you are agitated or struggling. Talk it out.

- Journaling can be a very cathartic way to deal with your emotions at this time.

- You have control over the situation and can control your health and weight.

- By focusing on your health and well-being, you will come out of the menopause far healthier than when you went into it.

Conclusion

And there we have it!

We have now reached the end of the book, and by this point, I hope you are feeling uplifted and more positive than you were at the beginning.

The menopause comes to all women. There is no escaping or avoiding it, but you can navigate your way through it and emerge with a smile on your face and a super-positive attitude.

I have said it before — the menopause does not define you as a woman. It does not give any value or take it away, it merely is a process which we all go through at this time in our lives and may cause some discomfort for some time. It is important to remember that you CAN handle this, just as you have handled everything else that life has thrown at you so far.

Add the menopause to your list of experiences which made you much stronger, because I promise you, by focusing on your health and well-being and learning to develop a more positive mindset, you will not waste one second of your time. There is no better way to react to a life change which may otherwise plunge you into the depths of worry and anxiety.

The main focus of this book is to help you avoid, lose and deal with menopausal weight gain. This is one of the most common effects of the menopause and it can be extremely challenging to deal with. Not only are you trying to handle all the other symptoms that are coming your way, but you are now noticing that your clothes are tighter and your body is changing shape. This has a way of knocking your self-confidence as well as changing the way you see yourself in the mirror.

Your weight does not define you either, but if you are a healthy weight and you like the way you look, your confidence will soar. Life is so much better when we are confident and happy with ourselves. That does not mean we need to be super-skinny; it means we need to be happy and healthy, that is it.

The advice I have given you in this book is all focused towards managing menopausal weight gain whilst handling the other symptoms. Many menopausal symptoms tend to wind into each other, such as sleep deprivation causing weight gain and mood changes. Low mood can affect weight gain because it is far easier to reach for something high in sugar when you are feeling down. Hormones can make you put on weight, but they can also affect your sleep and mood. The symptoms cause a vicious cycle, and this needs addressing. When you do that, you will notice benefits in various parts of your life no matter what your sole aim is.

By focusing on your health and well-being, you can make positive changes and dedicate yourself to leading a healthy lifestyle rather than following a random fad diet that is far too restrictive to be successful or manageable. You will notice that you will lose weight, feel great, have more energy, sleep better and feel more confident because of it. Therefore, the menopause could be the best time of your life if you allow it, and not a time which is entirely at the mercy of unrelenting hormones.

All that is left for me to do now is to wish you good luck. Be sure to take in every single piece of advice I have given you and please do not discount the idea of reaching out to other women going through the same experiences as you.

People around you can offer you plenty of safety, support and comfort. You should not have to deal with any challenging experience in life alone.

Our lives as women mean a constant change of events which lead towards a new life cycle. You are born, you release your first egg and start to menstruate, you have a monthly period for 30 or more years, you may have children, you may not, and then — just like that — Mother Nature decides that you have become too comfortable and she shakes things up a little.

When the storm is over, because at times it may feel like a storm, you will look back and be glad that you focused on the positive elements and protected your health for the many fun-filled years you have ahead of you.

I have given you a lot of information, but if you take anything from this book, I want it to be these key points:

- The menopause is the point at which you stop ovulating and stop releasing eggs.

- The period before the menopause begins is called the perimenopause. During this time, you may notice some symptoms, including irregular, light, or heavy periods.

- The main symptoms of the menopause include weight gain, hot flushes, night sweats, irritability, trouble sleeping and fatigue.

- Weight gain during the menopause can be a very troublesome issue for many women. During this time, visceral fat around the mid-section and abdomen is gained and it can be harder to lose than before.

- Hormonal imbalance during menopause is causing many changes inside your body.

- Not sleeping well affects your weight and contributes to low mood, trouble concentrating, and an increased risk of developing severe health issues in later life. Focusing on sleep quality is vital.

- By making sensible life choices and deciding to focus on your health and well-being, you can overcome many menopausal symptoms and reduce menopausal weight gain as a direct consequence.

- To focus on your health, you need to have a balanced, healthy diet and be physically active.

- Like many women, you may feel less attractive while going through the menopause but focusing on your health will help restore your confidence and radiance.

- The menopause is not a full stop to your active years, it is simply a process that you are going through for a while before entering a different stage of life.

- Seek out help and support from other women going through the same thing as you and be sure to talk to your nearest and dearest too.

- The menopause will end. It is not a cycle that is always going to be in your life.

- Remember, you are a strong woman, you are a warrior and you have got this!

There is never a better time than now to make a fresh start and take control of your health and your life. Be nice to yourself — do not wait another moment!

I wish you all the best!

Lots of love xx

Silvana

FREE YOURSELF FROM HOT FLUSHES AND NIGHT SWEATS

The Essential Guide to a Happy and Healthy Menopause

By Silvana Siskov

Introduction

The menopause is a challenging stage in a woman's life.

Some women have an easier time than others, but most women struggle at one point or another. There is a range of common symptoms during the menopause, and without a doubt, hot flushes and night sweats are up there as the most commonly experienced ones.

It is easy to assume that the menopause is a natural process; therefore, you just have to "put up" with the symptoms and wait for the storm to pass. But these days women do not have to let the menopause to control them. There are many approaches to take that can reduce the effects that menopausal symptoms have on your life. Very often, making small changes to your lifestyle can be enough to take the edge off the severity of troublesome symptoms you experience and allow you to go about your life more easily.

The aim of this book is to help you understand the reasons behind the most common menopausal symptoms, and then talk you through the ways you can reduce their effect on your life. You will discover that the majority of the symptoms can be reduced by focusing on a healthier approach to life. This would include cutting down on smoking and reducing alcohol intake, consuming a healthy diet packed with clean, fresh produce and a variety of vitamins and minerals, doing your best to get enough sleep, and including more exercise in your lifestyle. Many symptom treatment methods are often interlinked, so focusing on a healthier life overall will give you a head start in coping with several troublesome menopausal symptoms.

Overhauling your lifestyle may not be necessary. Perhaps you already exercise regularly, but you need to focus on your diet a little more. Maybe you do not drink or smoke, but you need to learn to find the time to exercise. People live their lives in many different ways, though there are healthy changes every woman can make to her lifestyle which can have far-reaching effects on her health and well-being, as well as her management of her menopausal symptoms.

Finding the time to exercise does not need to take a massive chunk out of your day. It can be just 20 to 30 minutes in the morning or during the evening. Eating a healthier diet and learning to cook, instead of ordering takeaways, is not too hard to achieve when you change your mindset and take on a new approach to dieting, and in this book I will show you how to do that. It can even save you money and be an enjoyable experience.

Focusing on health and well-being is your number one route towards a healthy and happy menopause.

Throughout this book, you will discover the role of hormones and how they affect you. I will give you information on why menopausal symptoms occur and what to do about them. Knowledge is power, and understanding what is going on in your body during this time of your life will provide you with the confidence to reduce the effects of its symptoms and alleviate any worries you may have.

In the first chapter of this book, I will give you some general information about the menopause to help you understand what is going on inside your body. Then, I will talk about the main symptoms and why they happen. You will see a recurring theme throughout this chapter and learn the leading cause of every symptom you experience.

There are over 30 menopausal symptoms, but it is worth remembering that not every woman is going to have the full list of symptoms that the menopause can bring.

By understanding why you experience particular symptoms and learning how to reduce them, you are giving yourself the best possible chance of achieving a healthier and happier experience. You may also be able to pass on your newly acquired knowledge to friends and family members who are also going through the menopause.

The remainder of the chapters will be dedicated to investigating specific common symptoms, exploring why the menopause happens and providing practical advice on how to reduce its effects naturally, wherever possible. I will also explain about hormone replacement therapy (HRT), a hot topic among women approaching and going through the menopause. HRT is a contentious subject and the one that you need to fully understand if you want to take advantage of its benefits — if you choose to do so.

It is a good idea to read through every symptom guide, because even if you are not dealing with it right now, it does not mean you will not in the future, and besides, focusing on optimal health is never a bad thing.

The menopause is very challenging, and at times you will be tired, you will be stressed out, and you will feel down. However, this book will give you the information you need to overcome those effects and feel far better as a result. There is no need to struggle alone and there is no need to assume that you just have to deal with it yourself. There is a lot of help out there. You will simply need to look for it, and in some cases, just ask for it.

The advice contained within this book will give you back the power to deal with this challenge you are faced with. You can then shape your response to the menopause in any way you see fit, owning your menopause, rather than allowing the menopause to own you.

Chapter 1

The Menopause Explained

Welcome to the first chapter!

The fact that you have read the book to this point means that you are interested in learning more about the menopause, how to deal with the symptoms, and how to reduce their impact on your life.

Before we delve into the symptoms and how to handle them better, I must give you some background information. You probably already know a little about what the menopause is, why it happens, and the types of things that can occur during this time. However, it is unlikely that you know it all. That is where this chapter is going to help you out.

In the following chapter, I will dive deep into the main menopausal symptoms and explain why you may experience them by exploring what is going on inside your body to cause them. But for now, let's look at what is going on inside your body generally at this time. Remember, knowledge is power!

Hormones and Their Key Role

If you are wondering why you are feeling hot, cold, sweaty, tired, anxious, agitated, or why you cannot sleep, it is mainly because of your hormones. Hormones are the thing that women have been battling with since day one.

When we are young, usually in our teens, our body prepares us for the ability to reproduce, and at this time, we experience our first major hormonal shift. As young women, we develop breasts, our hips widen, and we start our menstrual cycle. Each girl experiences this period of growing up and becoming a woman in her own way and in her own time.

Later, when we reach a certain age, our genetic matter is no longer at its prime to reproduce, so our bodies decide that it is time for us to stop procreating. Due to hormonal shifts that become more pronounced over time, our bodies are no longer able to carry a new life through pregnancy and safe delivery.

During this time, our hormones experience a significant change that might impact not only on our physical health, but also on our mental and emotional health. Therefore, it is vital to incorporate nutrition, physical activity, and even potentially a talking therapy to offer us well-being and emotional support through this period.

The power of hormones is enormous! Everything about how the body operates is connected to the delicate balance of hormone production. If you give your body the nutrition, activity, sleep, and peace of mind that it needs, it is designed to provide you with health in return. You get back what you put in!

The fluctuation of hormones during the menopausal phase might disrupt your body, causing a difference in your weight and affecting sleep patterns and your sex drive, among other factors. This is natural, normal and safe, and it does not have to be unbearable. However, if your hormones are confused because of regular yo-yo dieting and environmental disruptors, the changes you experience will be unnatural and will likely feel uncomfortable and perhaps cause some lasting damage too. Significant weight gain, particularly around your mid-section, unpredictable hot flushes, mood swings, and other symptoms of menopause, can be tempered when your body finds its natural balance again.

As you become older, your body creates increasingly lower amounts of female hormones, and as a result, the menopause begins. Here are the three main hormones which gradually diminish with age, causing you to experience menopausal symptoms:

- Oestrogen

- Progesterone

- Testosterone

Testosterone is a male hormone, but women also produce it and need it in small amounts.

As I have already mentioned, hormones are extremely powerful, which is why they have such a significant effect on some women and the way they feel. Hormones control a considerable number of functions within the body and they can lead to the development of certain conditions.

For instance, you may be at risk of developing osteoporosis in later life because of less oestrogen. Lack of oestrogen might make your bones weak and less flexible. You may also feel far less like having sex with your partner because you have less testosterone in your body, affecting the way you think, feel, and your general libido. Changes in hormones can also cause you to gain weight in specific areas during the menopause, usually around the midriff and abdomen.

The reduction of these critical hormones is the reason you are going through this change in life and why you might be feeling like you are going through hell.

Menopause may be a fact of life for all women, but it does not have to be a tragic health condition that is unavoidable. Normal and average do not necessarily correspond to natural or healthy, and there is a way to navigate through the menopause without having your entire life disrupted. Thankfully, we are going to talk about that in much more detail as we move through the book.

When Does the Menopause Happen?

If you search for the definition of the menopause, you will find something along the lines of "ceasing of menstruation". That means that your periods come to an end, and your body no longer releases an egg every month. You no longer bleed because you are not pregnant, and you no longer can become pregnant naturally. The good news is that you no longer have to deal with period cramps and other rather annoying symptoms that you have experienced for the last 30 or so years.

The menopause is a slow and steady process and often begins from around the age of 45 to 50 on average. However, you should not use those ages as a hard and fast guideline, because every woman is different. Some women start going through it much later, and others experience it much earlier.

There is a theory that women generally follow the pattern from their mothers. If your mother went through the menopause at the age of 45, for example, you would do the same. However, there is no concrete evidence to back this up. It is sometimes useful to look at your family history to predict the behavior of your genes, but in this instance, it might not be helpful. You can have a family of two sisters, one of them may follow the mother's pattern, whilst the other may be far younger or far older when her menopause begins. This has certainly been the case with my family.

The period before your menopause properly begins is called the perimenopause. This roughly translates to "around the menopause", so the time leading up to the actual point when you stop menstruating properly. During the perimenopausal stage, you might have a whole myriad of different symptoms. You will probably still have a monthly period, although sporadically, heavily or lighter than usual, and experience a range of other things that often fall into the perimenopausal "normal" range. It is not unusual for a woman's periods to become lighter, heavier, more irregular, more frequent, vary from spotting to heavy bleeding, and then back again. It is almost impossible to predict a pattern for your periods.

The perimenopause can last up to 10 years or so before the menopause is established. This is when you stop releasing eggs and stop menstruating. At this point, you are no longer fertile and can no longer become pregnant naturally. Symptoms can continue for another 10 years, although in most cases they will not be as severe. Remember, these are general patterns and must be heeded with caution, as every woman is different.

You should consider yourself as being through the menopause, i.e. postmenopausal, after you have not had a period at all for one year and are over the age of 50. If you are under the age of 40, you will need to be clear of periods for two years solidly, to be considered postmenopausal.

What About Premature Menopause?

If you go through the menopause before the age of 40, you are classed as having a premature menopause. It is thought that around 5% of women go through the menopause early, therefore falling into this premature bracket.

Understandably, premature menopause can be extremely upsetting for a woman, especially if she still hopes to have a family or extend the family she already has. There is no reliable indicator of whether a woman is likely to go through the menopause early; again, it could be that if her mother did, she would be more likely to follow suit, but this has not been proven.

There are some risk factors for having premature menopause, including:

- Women who suffer from chromosomal problems, e.g. Turner syndrome

- Women who suffer from autoimmune conditions (in rare cases however)

- Genetic – Again, if a female member of your close family went through premature menopause, you may be more likely to do so, but not certainly

- Cancer treatments, such as chemotherapy or radiotherapy, may cause premature menopause for some women

- Women who have had surgery to remove one or both ovaries

Premature menopause is sometimes called premature ovarian failure. The symptoms are the same as those experienced by an "average aged" menopausal woman. If you do go through premature menopause, you will probably be advised to take HRT (hormone replacement therapy), and this is something I will discuss in more detail a little later.

The Menopause is a Personal Deal

There is no denying that the menopause can be a challenging time for some women. On the other hand, some women sail through it and barely notice anything. It is a very personal deal and as a result, you should never compare your symptoms with a friend or a family member and then feel like there is something wrong with you if they do not match up.

Many women struggle with the fact that going through the menopause means that they are getting older. We cannot stop time, and getting older comes to us all, men included. So yes, the menopause is a sign of aging, but it is also a process that a woman's body needs to go through, and this does not make you any less attractive, or less feminine, or less powerful, or any less of a woman. If anything, it might even make you more of a woman, because you have taken on the ups and downs of the menopause and come out on top!

The menopause has the power to affect a woman's confidence in different ways; it can affect how you feel about yourself, your future, your appearance, and depending upon the age at which you go through the menopause, it might even mean that you have to come to terms with the fact that you are no longer able to carry a child of your own. The good news is that confidence can be built back up over time and a large part of handling the menopause and its symptoms is down to learning about the psychological and emotional effects.

Never be afraid of reaching out to those around you and talking about how you feel. If that is a little too close to home for you, find support in women your age, perhaps through social media or community support groups. You do not have to go through the menopause alone, and there is a lot of help and support out there if you reach out and ask.

This is your journey and one you should embrace as your own. In the rest of this book I will go into detail about some of the most common menopausal symptoms you might experience such as hot flushes, night sweats, lack of sex drive, headaches, etc., and give you plenty of advice on not only how to understand them, but also how to take them on and win!

Key Points

- The menopause happens to every woman. This is the time when periods stop, due to the ovaries no longer releasing eggs.

- The start of the menopause is called the perimenopausal period and can begin at any time between 45 to 50 years old.

- Some women experience premature menopause, which means they begin the menopause before the age of 40.

- The menopause is established when a woman has not had a period for one full year if she is over 50.

- If you experience the menopause in your forties or earlier, you would need to be clear of periods for two years to be considered menopausal.

- The postmenopausal period (after you have reached the menopause) can still cause symptoms, and these may last up to 10 years in some cases.

- Menopausal symptoms are caused by dwindling hormone levels, namely oestrogen, progesterone and testosterone.

- The menopause can affect a woman's self-confidence, as well as causing troublesome or upsetting symptoms.

- The menopause is unique for each woman and can create different issues for each of us.

Chapter 2

An Overview of Common Menopausal Symptoms

Now you know what the menopause is and why it happens. It is time to move on to the very crux of this book — the symptoms you might experience, why you might experience them, and what you can do to reduce their impact upon your life.

There is a range of different symptoms which many women experience during this time. Sometimes the symptoms are more prevalent during the perimenopause, whilst other women notice far more symptoms during the actual menopause itself. Even after menopause has been established, e.g. in the postmenopausal period, it is entirely normal to have some of the symptoms for up to around 10 years afterwards. There is no hard and fast rule to adhere to here, and it is partly about going with the flow and understanding what is going on inside your body and allowing nature to do what it needs to do.

You might feel as though you have zero control and that you are at the mercy of your hormones. I understand that. But believe me, you have more say in this than you realise; you can reduce the severity of most symptoms by changing your lifestyle and by thinking about different treatment methods.

Every Woman is Different

It is important to mention that every woman is different. Just because your friend, mother, sister, or anyone else experiences one particular symptom, that does not mean you are bound to. You might have a totally different set of symptoms from them. Your symptoms could be more severe or significantly less severe. You are a unique individual, and that means that your symptoms and your menopause might be slightly different or very different as a result.

Comparing your menopausal journey against another woman is not always useful because it can cause anxiety and worry if your experience is different, but the truth is that you are just going through your menopausal journey in your own unique way. Of course, if you are worried about something or if your symptoms become difficult to handle, you should definitely reach out to your doctor or another health professional to seek clarity and reassurance.

In the next chapter, we will talk about a few medical routes you could take, such as HRT, but for now, let's focus on the possible symptoms that may come your way, or in some cases, may not. We are going to look at why they are possible during this time and you will quickly see a pattern emerging; hormones are responsible for many ups and downs that you experience.

The Importance of Understanding What is Happening to Your Body

Before we get onto the specifics, there is one other thing you need to know: You have to know what is going on inside your body to understand how to deal with it in a healthy way. When you do not know why something is happening, it is easy to worry over it. You might start panicking whenever you experience it, even though it could be a common menopausal symptom and not something that should trigger anxiety. Worrying can further compound the symptoms you are experiencing. It is far better to arm yourself with knowledge and understand your body better as a result of it.

You can empower yourself by learning about the common symptoms and understanding why they are happening. Only then can you take control of the menopause.

It is essential to understand that sudden changes in your body temperature, sleepless nights, mood swings, brain fogs, and terrible headaches, can be put down to your hormones. Though you might not be directly aware of them, hormones have great power and the ability to change the way you think, act, and feel.

You may have found that your emotions or mood have not been taken seriously in the past and you have probably heard phrases like "oh, she's just hormonal", or "it's her hormones again." I find it disrespectful to hear these things, and I know that many women struggle to accept these sorts of comments. Hormones have the power to affect our physical, emotional, and mental health, whilst causing a myriad of symptoms which are very hard to connect.

To create a significant difference in your health and well-being, it is crucial to focus on lifestyle changes to make things easier for you. I am not saying that all your symptoms will suddenly disappear, but improving your health will likely reduce the impact of menopausal symptoms on your life, and some of those symptoms will gradually fade and will not return. When you focus on healthy living and start looking after your body, you will notice many positive changes happening to you on a physical, emotional, and psychological level. This is something we are going to talk about in far more detail as we move through the book.

Common Menopausal Symptoms and Why They Happen

Now, we are going to start getting to the real heart of the matter — menopausal symptoms and why they happen to us in the first place. As I have already mentioned, understanding why you are experiencing a specific symptom will allow you to feel calmer about it and then work out ways to control and minimise it, or possibly even remove it altogether.

Right now, I want to give you an informational overview of many menopausal symptoms that you might be experiencing, as it is important to get a broad view of what is happening to you at this time in your life. Then we are going to break your knowledge down into more distinct groups so you can get a better understanding of the range of symptoms that menopause can bring your way. In the coming chapters of this book, the focus will be on one specific symptom at a time and divided into different ways to control it.

I suggest that you do not skip any parts of the book and read all the chapters. All of the symptoms that I am going to discuss are common menopausal symptoms. Even if you are not experiencing some of the symptoms, you might find a useful piece of information and advice in this book which could help you live a healthier life in general.

Did you know there are over 30 menopausal symptoms that women can experience? So, what are the most common menopausal symptoms? Here is the list:

- Weight gain, specifically around the abdomen and midriff

- Hot flushes

- Night sweats

- Mood changes and irritation

- Fatigue

- Hair loss

- Anxiety

- Reduced libido

- Vaginal dryness

- Weak bones

- Brain fog

- Changes to the menstrual cycle, which then stop completely

- Problems sleeping

- Palpitations

- Headaches

- Focus and concentration problems

- Increased frequency of UTIs

- Thyroid issues

Before you panic, yes, that is a long list, but it does not mean you are going to experience all of those symptoms. Some women do, some do not, some have a few, some have half or more. Again, you are a unique individual, so we do not know what symptoms you may or may not have to deal with. It would not be unusual to start with one set of symptoms and then develop several more along the way; some might dwindle and disappear, only to come back a few months or a few years later. There is no pattern and no way of predicting which symptoms you may experience. You can only go with the flow and address what is in front of you.

I want to spend some time now informing you about the thyroid and its effects on your body because there is a strong connection between the menopause and thyroid disorder.

The thyroid is a small gland that sits at the front of your neck, just under what we call the "Adam's apple". The reason for thyroid issues to be quite common during this time of your life is that the thyroid comes under lots of pressure, due to the hormonal imbalance in your body.

You see, all the hormones work together and affect each other continuously. The thyroid is part of the endocrine system and it creates and releases two specific types of hormones, thyroxine and triiodothyronine. Both hormones are essential for ensuring the healthy functioning of the cells inside your body, and these hormones are also affected by other hormones. You already know that oestrogen, progesterone, and testosterone are reduced as the menopause approaches. As a result, this can sometimes cause problems with your thyroid and the treatment might be required to regulate and balance the hormones created and secreted by the thyroid.

Thyroid disorder is a complex condition that requires input from your doctor. The way to diagnose it is by taking your blood sample. Your doctor might ask you for the TSH test, T4 test, T3 test, and thyroid antibody test. These tests can show how well your thyroid is performing or how badly. Depending on the results, you might be prescribed a medication.

Many thyroid problems symptoms are very similar to the menopausal symptoms, and lots of women might be suffering from issues related to their thyroid disorder, but may think it is down to the menopause instead. Here are the most common symptoms of a thyroid disorder:

- Feeling tired a lot of the time

- Forgetfulness

- Putting on weight or losing it without trying

- Anxiety

- Feeling too hot or too cold

- Aches and pains in the joints and muscles

- Irregular periods

- Hair loss

- Dry and itchy skin

- Low mood

- Problems with concentration

Do you see the similarity between these symptoms and the symptoms of the menopause? That is why so many women fail to reach out to get treatment for their thyroid. They feel it is a part of their menopausal journey. My advice is, listen to your body and reach out if you suspect there may be a problem. You know your body better than anyone else and you should tune in and listen to what it is telling you. If your doctor does not take what you are saying seriously and you are concerned that something is not quite right, push the issue and ask for more tests. You are well within your rights to do so.

I would like to share my story with you now. I suffered from ill health for about five years from my late thirties to the early forties. I felt tired, had trouble sleeping, and I was losing my hair. Eventually, my periods started to become irregular. During this time, I visited a doctor regularly, until I was diagnosed with an underactive thyroid, a condition where the thyroid gland does not produce enough hormones.

I was prescribed medication for this condition, which I will probably take for the rest of my life, but this did not stop my troublesome symptoms from affecting me. During the perimenopausal phase my problems continued. Having an underactive thyroid and going through the perimenopause at the same time, I was never quite sure which of my symptoms were caused by the thyroid issue and which ones were triggered by the perimenopause, as they share many common symptoms.

Research shows that low levels of oestrogen caused by the menopause can significantly affect the thyroid hormones, but there are also suggestions that thyroid disorder can cause the menopause to start early — around the age of 40. As you can see, there is a clear link between thyroid issues and the menopause.

Let's now examine each menopausal symptom in turn and work out exactly why they happen during this time of your life. Please note, advice for dealing with some of these symptoms will be given in the coming chapters. Consider this your "why" educational chapter, with more to come later on how to deal with these issues.

Weight Gain

Some women notice that during the menopause they put on weight really easily, and it usually settles around the abdomen and midriff. This is called visceral fat and it is hard to shift once it sets up home. It is also a dangerous type of fat because it settles around the major organs.

Apart from causing health issues, weight gain also affects the way a woman feels about herself, which further compounds the overall effects of the menopause itself. By reducing your weight, you can increase your confidence, looking and feeling great in the process.

I will not dwell too much on this particular problem here, but if you want to learn more, please check my other comprehensive book on this subject, *Beat Your Menopause Weight Gain: Balance Hormones, Stop Middle-Age Spread, Boost Your Health and Vitality*. The book is packed with hints and tips on reducing menopausal weight gain and feeling better about yourself from the inside out. You will learn all about why weight gain happens during the menopause, the hormones that cause it, and what you can do about your menopausal weight gain. The book is available on Amazon.

Hot Flushes and Night Sweats

Two of the most common symptoms of the menopause are, without a doubt, hot flushes and night sweats. Most women will experience these symptoms, although to varying degrees.

A hot flush can be described loosely as a feeling of heat that comes over you quickly and without warning. It starts in one place in the body (varying from person to person), and it spreads very quickly. It often goes as quickly as it comes. Some women might notice that their face becomes flushed at the same time, whilst others may show no outside appearance of feeling hot at all. Some women may also have palpitations at the same time.

Night sweats cause excessive sweating while you are asleep, and you may wake up soaking wet. Many women are forced to change their nightclothes and bedsheets. They are very similar to hot flushes. The main difference is they happen during sleep and they can wake you up. Again, night sweats can disappear as quickly as they came. After the night sweat ends, you might be left freezing cold and in need of an extra blanket.

Hot flushes and night sweats are caused by (surprise, surprise!) hormones. The decline in oestrogen and progesterone has a knock-on effect on the other hormones in the body, especially the thyroid hormones which regulate body temperature. As a result, you may experience these surges and drops in body temperature, before returning to normal.

Both of these issues can be embarrassing, but they can also be rather worrying if you are not sure what is going on. If your hot flushes cause you to have palpitations, you might start to develop anxiety and panic, believing that you are having a heart attack. Of course, you are not, and breathing slowly and deeply should allow your heart rate to return to normal. Women who are experiencing their first few hot flushes, perhaps with palpitations brought on as a result, can experience this worry because they are not sure what is happening. This will also increase their anxiety levels.

Mood Changes, Irritation and Anxiety

Most women will notice a change in their mood occasionally during the menopause. This may be more severe for some women than others. The feeling of wanting to snap at everyone and everything, feeling agitated and annoyed for no reason, and then perhaps feeling extremely down, are quite common.

Again, as with most symptoms, we need to look towards the decreasing level of oestrogen and progesterone within the body. It is very common for this to cause mood changes, depression in some cases, anxiety, and a general lack of energy. As your body adjusts to the lower oestrogen level, this should even itself out. If you are really struggling, do not struggle alone; reach out for help from your doctor and discuss your problems with them.

Reduced Libido and Vaginal Dryness

The reduction in the two female sex hormones can have a drastic effect on libido for some women. Many women notice that they feel far less bothered about sex during the perimenopausal period in particular.

These dwindling hormones can also lead to vaginal dryness which can cause discomfort and even pain during sex. Of course, this will also have a knock-on effect on how you feel about having intercourse and is likely to place it far down your priority list.

This may affect your relationship if you are in one, so you must communicate with your partner and let them know what is going on — they may take it personally and blame themselves for your lack of sexual desire.

Weak Bones

The menopause changes your body in many different ways, but as you age, you will most probably notice the changes in your body. As oestrogen levels drop, bone density levels drop along with it. This is because oestrogen helps to keep your bones strong, healthy and flexible, and the less oestrogen there is, the more chance you have of weakening bones, placing you at a higher risk of fractures and breaks.

Over time, you may develop a risk of osteoporosis, also known as brittle or weak bones. When this happens, it is far easier to fracture/break a bone than otherwise. However, just because you are going through the menopause, it does not mean this is necessarily going to happen; the risk of osteoporosis increases as you age in general, and there are things you can do to help protect against this. We will talk about that in far more detail as we move through the book, but most of it comes down to simple lifestyle changes and awareness of what a healthy lifestyle involves.

Changes to the Menstrual Cycle

Every woman experiences this particular symptom while approaching the menopause. By the end of the menopause your symptoms will have stopped completely, but in the years leading up to it, i.e. in the perimenopausal period, you will notice that your periods become irregular in terms of timing and/or flow. They may be lighter or heavier for a while, they will stop and then restart again, and will basically cause you a little bit of inconvenience.

The lowering of the two sex hormones means that your periods are not regular and are not within a pattern like they used to be. It is impossible to predict your periods during the perimenopausal stage because your hormones are playing havoc with them.

Problems Sleeping

The whole cocktail of problems and hormonal imbalance that the menopause brings can easily disrupt a woman's sleep pattern and make it harder to get a good night's shut eye.

As oestrogen and progesterone decline, hot flushes and night sweats begin, anxiety and low mood may start, can make it very hard to either get to sleep in the first place or stay asleep for long. The more sleep deprived you become, the worse you feel the following day. This is one of the reasons why some menopausal women feel quite tired and drained most of the time.

Palpitations and Headaches

You may be tired of hearing "it's because of your hormones." However, hormones are responsible for causing the risk of palpitations and headaches.

Palpitations during menopause are often harmless, but you should seek medical help if they are too frequent or you feel worried about them. For the most part, palpitations occur during a hot flush, due to your body temperature surging.

Headaches are also likely to be frequent at this time, again due to hormonal imbalance.

However, if you are worried about your heart palpitations and recurring headaches or migraines, you must check them out with your doctor. There are many other reasons for these symptoms to occur, and they may not be brought on by the menopause only. It is important to do a proper examination if they are very regular or causing you significant discomfort.

Focus and Concentration Problems

Due to your hormones being in decline, you might experience brain fog during the perimenopausal period. You have no doubt heard about the "baby brain" that new mothers get, which is down to hormones at that time. The same goes for the trouble concentrating that you might experience during the perimenopausal period.

If the menopause keeps affecting your mood significantly, causing you anxiety and depression, that could also be the reason for your focus and concentration issues.

Increased Frequency of UTIs

As this is one of the less common menopausal symptoms, I will not allocate a chapter to this particular issue, but it is worth discussing it briefly in this section. UTIs (urinary tract infections) or water infections, as they are more commonly known, may become more frequent during the menopause for some women. Again, this is down to oestrogen levels declining.

As oestrogen declines, the urethra changes a little. This is the tube that takes urine from the bladder and outside as you urinate. It depends how this decreased oestrogen level affects your particular urethra, but for some women this can be enough to lead to a higher risk of UTIs. They are not particularly pleasant, as you will know if you have ever had one. Most importantly, they can easily be treated by your doctor.

In this chapter, I have highlighted the most common menopausal symptoms, along with a quick rundown of why they are likely to be happening to you. You will notice one very clear pattern in all of them, which is a decrease in female sex hormones as the primary cause.

This is the main reason for all menopausal symptoms occurring, and the power those hormones have over your entire body can be quite startling if you are not informed of what is going on. Now you know exactly the reason for your symptoms, and that should give you a certain amount of reassurance that you are going through an entirely normal process called the menopause. However, as I have mentioned a few times already, if you are at all worried, I advise you to speak to your doctor for reassurance, and further advice by doing some tests and getting to the bottom of your troublesome symptoms.

Key Points

- Every woman is unique and might experience different menopausal symptoms from those of their friends or family members.

- There are several common menopausal symptoms. However, the most common include hot flushes, night sweats, weight gain, mood changes, anxiety, vaginal dryness and low libido, bone weakness, sleep issues, and problems concentrating.

- It is important to get familiar with the most common menopausal symptoms and understand why they occur.

- Hot flushes and night sweats are the most complained about menopausal symptoms, and these can also cause issues with sleep.

- Changing your lifestyle can help with many menopausal symptoms.

- If you are not sure if a symptom you experience is harmless or not, or if you are struggling with the severity of your symptoms, visit your doctor. You should always check things out if something is troubling you and causing you discomfort.

Chapter 3

A Word About HRT

Most women who go to see their doctor about menopausal symptoms are given the option of hormone replacement therapy (HRT). Some women are totally against it, others are open to it, and some of them are not quite sure. It is important to get as much information on the subject as possible before deciding whether this is the right treatment for you.

HRT is not a blanket approach to the menopause. You do not have to take it, you might not even need to take it, perhaps you are not suitable for it, but many women are offered it. It is essential to know the facts about HRT and make an informed choice that is personal to you.

There are many benefits to taking HRT, but there are also some side effects and risks. If you choose not to go with

HRT, there are a few alternative options that you may want to consider. This will be discussed later on in this chapter.

Because HRT is a standard menopausal treatment and your doctor is likely to offer it to you for treating your symptoms, an entire chapter in this book is dedicated to this subject to give you the necessary information that you need to know.

HRT is given as a medical treatment to women going through the menopause (if they choose to take it) to help relieve the menopausal symptoms. As the name suggests, the drug replaces some of the hormones that have been reduced due to the menopause. If a woman is having an incredibly hard time with one or more symptoms, HRT may help to relieve them.

Most women can take HRT, but as with anything, there are a few anomalies. You might not be able to take HRT if you have any history or a family history of breast, ovarian or endometrial cancer, blood clots, or if you have liver disease or any problems with high blood pressure (hypertension). If you do have blood pressure problems, your doctor will need to stabilise it with medication before considering whether to prescribe HRT. Always listen to your doctor's advice on suitability and be sure to consider your decision very carefully. You do not have to make a decision immediately; you can go away and think about it first.

The Benefits and Side Effects of HRT

The main benefit of HRT is that it can reduce troublesome menopausal symptoms and therefore allow you to go through the menopause with far less trouble. This does not mean that you will not have any symptoms at all, but they will be far fewer and more manageable.

It is still a good idea to make lifestyle changes if you are taking HRT, because focusing on your overall health and well-being by following a healthy diet, doing regular exercise and establishing a healthy sleep routine as you become a little older is always recommendable regardless. This will also help you to become more mindful of what constitutes positive and healthy versus what does not. It is easy to fall into unhealthy patterns and habits as we go through life, so this is an excellent opportunity to look at the rights and wrongs and readjust.

HRT has always had a slightly dubious reputation. This is because, whilst it is a very effective treatment for many women, it does have a few risks attached to it. The benefits are often thought to outweigh the downsides, but it is something that has to be decided on carefully if you are interested in trying this drug. I recommend you speak to your doctor, who will weigh up the pros and cons with you and find the best type for you (more on that shortly) and ultimately decide whether or not it is safe for you.

The main side effects of HRT include:

- Tender breasts

- Headaches

- Nausea

- Indigestion

- Bloating

- Vaginal bleeding

- Abdominal pain

- Leg cramps

If you do experience side effects when taking HRT, they are usually mild and they should even out after about three months of taking them. However, if you find the side effects too troublesome or they are worrying you, go to see your doctor and change the type you are taking or ask the doctor for an alternative. Remember, just because you are going through the menopause, does not mean that you have to take HRT. It is an option that is there for you if you want it.

If you do decide to take HRT, there is not an actual time frame on how long you can take it for, but your doctor will advise you on when you should stop.

Most women stop taking HRT after their menopausal symptoms have settled down. There is an increased risk of breast cancer linked to HRT, so this is something you have to bear in mind when it comes to deciding whether to start taking it and how long to take it for. You can choose to stop taking HRT whenever you want to, but it is a good idea to wean yourself off to check whether or not your menopause symptoms come back. If they do, you can continue taking it for a bit longer.

Different Types of HRT

There are a few different types of HRT, and your doctor will advise you on the best one for you.

Here are the main types:

- *Combination* – e.g. a combination of both oestrogen and progesterone, to replace what you are naturally lacking. This can be done through tablets, skin patches, gels, pessaries, rings, or a vaginal cream.

- **_Oestrogen-only_** – Women who have had a hysterectomy in the past, e.g. no longer have a womb, can take oestrogen only HRT, and again, this is available in different formats, such as tablets, gels, etc.

There are different ways to take HRT. You might start on a lower dose, and then it might get increased at the later stage. You may even be prescribed to take oestrogen continually and then progesterone added in for a few weeks and then repeat the cycle; it depends on your body and what it needs. Your doctor will advise you about this.

Possible Alternatives to HRT

Of course, you might not want to take HRT and that is fine. There are a few alternatives you could look into and again, it is up to you whether you go with them or not.

Many women stick to lifestyle changes only and it works very well for them. We are all different, so make sure you choose a method of working your way through the menopause that suits you and your needs. Your friend might swear by one particular method, but you might try it and find no relief whatsoever.

The main alternatives to HRT, aside from lifestyle changes alone, include:

- Tibolone

- Antidepressants

- Clonidine

- Complementary therapies

Tibolone

You will find Tibolone marketed under the name "Livial" and this is a drug that your doctor has to prescribe. Tibolone is similar to HRT in that it puts back the hormones you are lacking, and it is thought to be particularly useful for hot flushes, mood problems, and reduced libido in particular.

Only postmenopausal women can take Tibolone and it is designed to help with the dwindling menopausal symptoms as they can last for many years after the menopause is established. There are side effects (abdominal and pelvic pain, tender breasts, vaginal discharge and itching) and there is an increased risk of breast cancer and strokes, so discuss this option carefully with your doctor beforehand.

Antidepressants

Some women find that antidepressants can help them with their menopausal symptoms, especially hot flushes and low mood. Whilst antidepressants are not licensed for menopausal symptom use, they are thought to be useful, so it is up to you to look at this possibility.

We all know that antidepressants can have some unpleasant side effects, such as agitation, nausea, reduced libido, dizziness, and anxiety. These side effects usually reduce and disappear after three months of use but again, you need to discuss this with your doctor if you are struggling.

Clonidine

Clonidine is used for treating high blood pressure, drug withdrawal, and attention deficit hyperactivity disorder (ADHD).

For women struggling with hot flushes and night sweats, in particular, Clonidine could be very useful. As Clonidine is not associated with hormones, there is no increased risk of breast cancer to consider, and this appeals to many women. However, some women may not find this medication very effective for their menopausal symptoms.

Clonidine usually takes around two weeks to a month to show significant effects and can cause tiredness, constipation, dry mouth, and even depression. Again, speak to your doctor if you think Clonidine might help you, or you are struggling with its side effects.

Alternative Medicine

I want to point out that most alternative medicines are not backed up by scientific evidence, yet many women do try them, so I want to put a few ideas here for you to consider for yourself.

You will find a few products on the shelves of health stores or online that are reputed to help with specific menopausal symptoms, the main ones being:

- Evening primrose oil

- St John's wort

- Ginseng

- Black cohosh

- Angelica

Most of these are reputed to reduce hot flushes in particular, but the problem is that the complementary and alternative industry is not regulated in the same way as the pharmaceutical industry. That means you can purchase a product believing it is high-quality, but the ingredients either are not good quality, or you are not recommended to take the right dose.

I will not give you recommendations on which companies are the best sources of high-quality products, as it depends on what is suitable in the country you reside in, but I suggest you do your research on this.

When searching on the internet, it is worth mentioning that it is a good idea to spend a little more money and find a quality product with plenty of positive reviews, rather than opting for a lower cost one. Please note that taking a supplement with the brand name does not mean it is a good quality supplement. It is also important to remember that when taking a cheap supplement, you often get what you pay for.

This chapter has given you a few ideas on how you might like to treat your menopausal symptoms medically. But you do not have to do this, and you might prefer to stay with natural methods via changing your diet and adding in a few healthy lifestyle measures. The choice is yours, but it is essential to look at different options when searching for the best solution.

It is vital to get the information you need from reliable sources to choose how to approach your menopausal journey based on your own informed decision.

The rest of this book focuses on managing menopausal symptoms naturally instead of using supplements or medications.

Dealing with my menopausal symptoms naturally was my preferred method and when my doctor offered me HRT, I refused to take it.

Prioritising a healthy lifestyle will affect your hormones and make a positive difference in your life as a menopausal woman. You can do many things to help yourself, and there are numerous methods you can apply to help you live a healthy and symptom-free life.

Key Points

- HRT stands for hormone replacement therapy, and it replaces hormones that are at a lower level due to approaching the menopause.

- Not all women use HRT, but it is an option for you if you want to take it.

- There are benefits to taking HRT, but there are also side effects and these need to be discussed with your doctor and weighed up.

- The final decision over whether you take HRT or not is yours, but it is not suitable for some women and your doctor will inform you if you fall into that category.

- HRT does not completely take away your menopausal symptoms, but it may help reduce their severity, therefore making the menopause more manageable for you.

- Some of the most common HRT side effects include tender breasts, headaches, nausea, indigestion, abdominal pain and vaginal bleeding.

- There are several types of HRT and a few alternatives to explore with your doctor.

- Alternative medicine should be discussed with your doctor before you consider using them.

Chapter 4

Battling Hot Flushes and Night Sweats

As I have already mentioned, two of the most common menopausal symptoms that affect most women at this time of life are hot flushes and night sweats. Hot flushes, in particular, are incredibly annoying, can feel embarrassing and uncomfortable, and they tend to come out of nowhere.

On the other hand, night sweats can cause many health issues as they prevent you from having a good night's sleep. Lack of sleep can negatively impact your health causing you to have a low mood, increased irritability, and difficulty concentrating. It can also affect your appetite, which could lead you towards putting on weight.

You will quickly come to see that most symptoms affect one another.

In an earlier chapter of this book, I talked about the fact that hot flushes and night sweats are both caused by an imbalance of hormones, affecting the thyroid, which regulates body temperature. A few of the treatment methods I talked about in the last chapter can be very useful for hot flushes in particular, but even if you go down the medical route, e.g. HRT or one of the alternatives I mentioned, you are likely to need to make a few changes to your routine too. Handily, it is relatively easy to do it once you know how, and the effects can be far-reaching.

Lifestyle Changes to Reduce Hot Flushes and Night Sweats

There are a few things you can do to reduce hot flushes and night sweats, and it is not impossible to eliminate them completely. Soon we will look at the importance of a healthy diet and how it links to this particular symptom.

First, let us focus on to general changes you can make to your lifestyle and routine so that these symptoms become a fleeting issue rather than a chronic problem that stays with you for a long time and makes you feel miserable.

Wear Light Clothing

You need to be warm if it is sub-zero outside, but when you are in the house or at work, try wearing light clothing if possible, and avoid synthetic materials that hold in the heat and make you feel a little sweaty. Lightweight cotton is an excellent fabric to keep you cool.

When you go to bed, choose only light clothing and think about breathable materials for your bedding too. The more cool air that can move around you, the more comfortable you will feel. Sure, this will not stop you from having these symptoms, but it will reduce their severity and help make you more comfortable in general. When a hot flush arrives, it will not be as burning hot, and after experiencing night sweats you might have less of a clammy feeling. These changes and improvements can be quite dramatic when you make the right adjustments.

Regulate the Bedroom Temperature

If night sweats are a big problem for you, regulating your bedroom temperature could help. Keep your bedroom as cool as you can, perhaps opening windows and using a fan to circulate air around the room. As before, stick to light and breathable fabrics for whatever you wear for bed and for the bedding itself. If you have air conditioning in your room, make use of it and set it on a moderate temperature.

This change can be difficult if your partner likes the room a little warmer, but you are going to have to have a conversation in that case and make them understand your position. There is bound to be some middle ground you can arrive at and if you are waking them up because you are bothered by hot flushes and night sweats, they might welcome this adjustment because it means they get a better night's sleep.

Sip on Cold Drinks

You might love tea and coffee, but drinking hot drinks will send your temperature up, and when this is already a problem, it will not help you.

Keep a jug of water or juice in the fridge filled with ice cubes and regularly sip on it. Or use an insulated mug to keep the contents chilled. By doing that, you are helping to keep your body temperature down and helping reduce hot flushes throughout the day. You are also staying hydrated, which is very important for overall health and well-being and will have a related effect on other troublesome symptoms, such as headaches.

Stop Smoking

Smoking is damaging for your health in general, but it could be making your hot flushes much worse. Studies suggest that quitting smoking decreases the risk of midlife hot flushes and showed that smoking could reduce oestrogen levels in the body, therefore increasing your risk of having a hot flush. This means that the more you smoke, the worse your flushes will be.

Make a healthy choice to stop smoking for the sake of your health, but also to reduce your hot flushes. The benefits of quitting smoking are tremendous for health and general well-being. If you need help to stop smoking, discuss this with your doctor, who may be able to refer you to a smoking cessation advisor. There are many methods that can help you quit smoking, including patches, meditation, and good old willpower. Whatever method you choose, quitting smoking will prove to be one of the best decisions you will ever make and will certainly affect many of the other symptoms you may be experiencing, in a very positive way.

Exercise Regularly

I am sure you are aware that exercise is good for your health. Exercising regularly is vital for your heart health, mood, and gives a myriad of other great benefits. But did you know that exercise might also help to reduce the severity and intensity of your hot flushes?

Studies show that exercising can benefit menopausal symptoms and the study done by Harvard medical school showed a 60% reduction in the frequency of hot flushes after experiencing an increased heart rate due to exercising.

I know that many women are familiar with the countless benefits of exercise, but did you know that doing too much exercise can be as bad for you as leading a sedentary lifestyle. "Why is this?" you may ask.

As I mentioned earlier, menopause decreases oestrogen levels, which is one of the main reasons for your hot flushes. Excess exercise can further lower your oestrogen. Also, too much exercise could put your body under stress which will increase your cortisol levels. Cortisol is a stress hormone and known to cause hot flushes. I suggest you look at the type of exercise you choose to do and the level you are going to perform your aerobic activity.

Moderation is the key, remember this. You do not need to pound the treadmill at the gym every single day; you simply need to get your heart rate up and sweat a little (ironic, right?). Your body will naturally regulate its own temperature, which will eliminate those irregularities.

By doing this, not only will you become fitter and healthier and your mood will improve, but you will also find that you have fewer hot flushes. Combining this with the other methods I have mentioned will give you a greater chance of success and help with a range of other symptoms that we are going to look at throughout the rest of the book.

Reduce Your Stress Levels

Stress is no good for your health, and it is one of the leading killers in today's society. Not only can it worsen your hot flushes and night sweats, but it can also prove to be fatal for your health when allowed to accumulate over a more extended period. It might sound drastic, but it is true. The more stress you allow into your life, the more cortisol your body will produce. Over a long period of time, this can lead to having far too much cortisol circulating around your body.

Cortisol is a stress hormone. When the raised cortisol level interacts with your female sex-hormones which are imbalanced due to the menopause, your hot flushes are likely to be more troublesome than ever before, along with an impending sense of doom and anxiety that stress tends to initiate.

Reducing stress is not easy, but there are ways you can do it. Try meditation, play a sport or exercise, focus on sleep and diet, and talk about whatever is bothering you. We tend to hold everything inside and allow stress to build and build, until we reach the point of no return.

Allowing stress to take over your life is no good for your health and it is no good for your hot flushes or night sweats either.

Stress management is a very real thing, so make sure you pay attention to changing your routine and make it a priority.

The Role of Diet

What you eat can affect your hot flushes and night sweats too. Certain foods are good for you and could have a beneficial effect on reducing the number of hot flushes and night sweats you are experiencing, and there are some which are best to avoid.

When you eat highly processed foods, rich in sugar or salt and unhealthy fats, then chemicals and hormones in your body change. This affects your menopausal symptoms and can increase the frequency and strength of the hot flushes you experience.

To prove the importance of a good diet with women experiencing hot flushes, a study done by medical anthropologist Margaret Lock in 1998 found that Japanese women suffered less hot flushes than women in the western world. This is thought to be down to a different kind of diet, which focuses more on fresh and clean foods, as opposed to the western-style diet rich in processed foods, high sugar content, and many synthetic ingredients.

Convenience foods were invented to help keep us sane and afloat in an increasingly busy world, but if we consider the toll it takes on our health, both physical and mental, it turns out they are far from convenient.

I understand that if you rarely cook food from scratch, the prospect of doing so regularly could be intimidating. But the more time you practice this skill, the more you handle vegetables, roots, and grains in their original forms, the more comfortable you will get with them.

If you want to reduce your hot flushes and night sweats, be sure to eat more of the foods on the "do" list and less of the ones on the "do not" list below.

Do list:

- ***Fresh fruit and vegetables*** – Not only are these far better for your health, but many researchers have found that a Mediterranean-style diet, i.e. a diet which is packed with fresh, whole foods, can help to reduce the number of hot flushes a woman experiences. Every additional serving of whole, nutrient-dense plants will have a positive impact on your health.

- **Whole-grains** – Again, these are a much healthier alternative to processed grains that can increase hot flushes and cause all manner of digestive issues. Stick to whole-grain versions of bread, rice, pasta, etc.

- **Soy** – There is some suggestion that soy products, such as soy milk, edamame beans and tofu, could help to reduce the number of hot flushes and night sweats a woman experiences in menopause. It is because the oestrogen from plants can regulate the hormones in your body and therefore reduce your symptoms as a result.

- **Flax seeds** – Flax seeds contain the healthy types of fat you need in your diet for overall health and well-being, and you can easily sprinkle these onto your morning porridge or your muesli, or just throw them into something you are baking. They are rich in plant oestrogen and they can balance hormone levels and drastically cut the number of hot flushes in many cases.

- **Strawberries** – Not only are they delicious, but strawberries are thought to reduce hot flushes. Again, it is down to the fact that they contain plant oestrogen. Besides, they are also high in Vitamin C, giving you an immune system boost and balancing out your hormones.

- **Healthy fats** – I have already mentioned flax seeds, but the healthy type of fat is an excellent addition to your diet if you want to reduce hot flushes and increase your general health and well-being. Omega-3 fatty acids are the best type to focus on here, and that means a good weekly intake of fatty fish, such as mackerel, sardines, etc. You can also get a fair amount of omega-3 fatty acids from leafy green vegetables, canola oil and soybeans.

Do not list:

- **Spicy foods** – Any food which causes your body temperature to rise is likely to bring on a hot flush, and foods that are high in spice content do exactly this. Avoid chillies as they contain capsaicin which dilates blood vessels and increases temperature.

Black pepper contains piperine, which does the same thing.

- **Alcohol** – Of course, everything in moderation, but alcohol is known to increase hot flushes for many women. Again, it dilates the blood vessels and makes hot flushes more likely. This does not happen to all women, but it is a fairly common effect. If you love your evening glass of wine, I suggest that you cut down and have it less frequently, or find an alcoholic beverage that affects you less.

- **Caffeine** – Opt for decaffeinated drinks rather than the full-on caffeinated versions as caffeine can make hot flushes worse. If you really cannot do without, try and let your coffee cool down before drinking it and limit your intake to one cup per day.

- **Sugar** – Many studies have found that women who have a high sugar diet tend to have more hot flushes. In that case, you need to cut down as much as you can, and of course, that will also help your overall health. It is recommended by WHO (World Health Organisation) that you should consume less than six teaspoons of sugar every day, so that is a good marker to aim for. If you have a sweet tooth, you might find this a tough habit to kick but try substituting your sweet treats for other healthier options, such as yogurt, fruit, and nuts. It can be done!

If you have not done it already, I advise you to visit bit.ly/menopause-healthy-recipes-2 and download *Healthy Eating for Menopause – Recipe Book*. It is packed with delicious recipes to support you on your menopause journey.

By making the right kind of lifestyle changes and watching what you eat, you might be able to reduce your hot flushes and night sweats down to a minimum; in some cases, you may be able to rid yourself of them completely. Just remember, by the time you are 50, you will have eaten more than 50,000 meals. That is a considerable tradition to contend with, so have patience with yourself. Start with one step at a time.

My Client Ronnie

I want to tell you about my client, Ronnie (the name has been changed, to respect the privacy of my client). When I first met her, she had just turned 50. Not only was she trying to overcome her weight loss issues, but fluctuations of hormones during the menopause also starting to overwhelm her.

Sleepless nights had never bothered her in the past, but the missing sleep suddenly made her days feel never-ending and an uphill battle. She used to have regular night sweats which kept her awake most nights. Even though she was constantly exhausted, she still could not sleep. This was an extremely frustrating experience for her.

She also struggled with hot flushes during the day. They did not help her comfort levels at all. In the most inopportune moments, she would overheat, leaving her soaked through with sweat in minutes. She found this unbearable at times.

Many women struggle with this experience, and there is nothing that can prepare us for it. But it is important to know that simple diet and lifestyle changes can often reduce the frequency and severity of these symptoms of menopause.

With plenty of encouragement and support, Ronnie made a few changes to her nutrition and the way she was eating. She also followed my advice on getting into habit of moving her body more often. Within a month, she was sleeping soundly enough to feel rested most days and when I asked her about her hot flushes, she could not even remember the last time she had them.

What she was really excited about, however, was the fact that she not only enjoyed her new, healthy meal plan, but she did not feel like she was on a diet. She was never hungry. Also, she was losing weight.

By focusing on her health, Ronnie was able to naturally help her body address the issues so many women struggle with — disordered eating and weight management. And she was learning to love her body in her early fifties because she had an entirely new lease on life that was completely unexpected.

Key Points

- Hot flushes and night sweats are the most common symptom with menopausal women, and they can be very annoying and upsetting.

- Hot flushes, in particular, can come and go quickly or stick around for longer.

- Hot flushes and night sweats can affect your sleep pattern and therefore make many of your other menopausal symptoms worse.

- Wear light clothing to bed and make sure your room temperature is not too hot.

- Smoking can make hot flushes worse, so work on quitting smoking to improve your general health and well-being.

- Regular exercise can reduce instances of hot flushes.

- Stress can also make hot flushes worse, so work on stress management.

- Diet plays a role in hot flushes, and there are several foods you should focus on and avoid to help hot flushes becoming a significant problem for you.

Chapter 5

The Mental Health Effects of the Menopause

The menopause does not just affect your body, but your mind too. Changes in your hormones can throw your emotions for a much unexpected turn and you may experience low mood, agitation, anxiety, stress, mood swings and low confidence.

While we would never say that it is "normal" to feel this way, some people would argue that it is normal for the menopause to be this way. Feeling depressed, anxious, agitated, etc. is often a result of the hormonal imbalance that is in charge of a woman's body during the menopause transition. Some women might feel that something far more worrying is going on when they experience these symptoms, but I can assure you that it is the hormones that affect your well-being. That is the power that hormones can have over you.

Nowadays, we are increasingly encouraged to talk about our mental health, which can only be a good thing. Almost everyone will experience low mood at some point in their lives, and if you have experienced this once or twice already, you will know that it is not something you will want to put up with. The truth is that you DO NOT have to just put up with feeling this way and there is plenty you can do to help yourself, or you can reach out and get help from others.

During this time of your life, seeking help to support your emotional and psychological needs might be necessary. This can be done in many different ways and some women choose to take supplements or medication, while others decide to go to talking therapies or join activities such as yoga or meditation.

Do not feel that because you are going through the menopause you simply have to just deal with the symptoms that are common for this time in a woman's life. Not doing anything about it is a fast track to a miserable menopause, which may go on for many years. I suggest you be proactive and work on making your life more comfortable. Remember, you are in the driving seat.

You have to decide where you are going and make sure that you get there safely.

In the following sections, I will give you many suggestions and plenty of guidance on the actions you can take to feel good about your body, and be positive about your life, so that the menopause will feel more like a light breeze rather than a hurricane blowing in your face at a speed of 150 miles per hour.

You Do Not Have to Suffer From Low Mood

The hormonal imbalance caused by the perimenopause and menopause itself can cause chaos on so many levels, but the effects can be the hardest to deal with as far as mental health is concerned. It is essential to talk to your family and friends as much as possible because perhaps they do not realise how you are feeling, and they do not understand why you might occasionally snap at them. They want to help and support you, but first, you need to open up and talk about how you are feeling. Having them on your side will certainly make things easier and will also reduce the chances of fallouts and arguments.

In the past, women have assumed that experiencing low mood, having difficulty concentrating and focusing, or suffering from anxiety, stress, and mood swings is something that is expected of middle-age women. But we do not live in those days anymore. Nowadays, we do not have to bear the symptoms of the menopause and there are lots of things we can do to reduce the severity of the symptoms.

Poor mental health can be caused by so many things, including the menopause, but not one of these causes is a good enough reason for feeling low or agitated or being constantly anxious. We talk so openly about our physical health, but we are still worried about opening up too much about our mental health. Why not make a pact with yourself that one good thing to come out of the menopause for you will be an openness about how you are feeling, a willingness to talk about things that upset you, and focusing on self-care? I think we could all do with more of that, whether we are going through the menopause or not.

Of course, the changes your body is going through can cause you to feel less confident, but remember that you are not less of a woman or less attractive because you are going through the menopause. You are not less worthy than before because of the changes you are going through, and not one stage of the menopause defines you as a woman. This can be difficult to accept when you are going through it, however that is where focusing on self-care comes into it. In many ways, when done in the right way, the menopause can increase your confidence, believe it or not. You will finally understand your body and your power as a woman.

The more you focus on looking after yourself; the mind, body, and soul, the more you will notice your self-confidence increasing. Also, the more you practice gratitude, the happier and healthier you will be — inside and out. New opportunities will come your way as a result of it all, and who knows where those new chances in life may take you.

How to Naturally Boost Your Feel-Good Factor

There are many ways you can practice self-care and make yourself feel better in the process. I am going to share some techniques with you that you can try without making a huge effort, but the effects will be substantial.

Many women feel that they do not deserve a little pampering and the time to focus on themselves. Some women feel guilty about having "me time". They feel as though they are being selfish because they are so used to dedicating their time and love to everyone else around them. It almost seems "wrong" to focus on themselves every now and then.

Here are some suggestions to help you give yourself a break and focus on your own needs instead of pleasing everybody else, i.e. your spouse, children, elderly parents, work colleagues, friends, etc. This is YOUR time and you need it — you deserve it!

Be Kind to Yourself

Be kind to yourself is my first suggestion. You are going through a change in your life and any change is sure to make you feel a little out of sorts. Make peace with that fact and accept that it is perfectly acceptable to feel that way.

Far too often women have been forced to simply "get on with it" as quietly as possible, but we are not in the 1800s anymore! We are allowed to talk about how we are feeling and make time for ourselves.

Self-care is vital during this time in your life. Be kind to yourself and do the things that make you happy. If you love to spend time having a warm bubble bath before bedtime or read a book, then do it. If you love going to the cinema and eating a bucket of popcorn to yourself, why not do it? (Occasionally, of course). If dancing is your thing, grab your dancing shoes! Whatever makes you feel good and gives you confidence, you need to do more of it, and take the time to really nourish your mind, body, and soul.

Everything in moderation should be your mantra. So, if you fancy having a piece of cake once per week, then do it. Moderation is key and will unlock the door to health and happiness. One piece of chocolate cake a week is not going to kill you, and one session in the gym with a personal trainer will not make you fit, slim and healthy. Distinguishing what is healthy and what is unhealthy for you is the key. And creating the balance using this knowledge is crucial.

Practice Positivity

I often hear women having a conversation with one another and discussing how the menopause is affecting their physical, mental and emotional state. I also hear them agree that it is normal for menopausal women to be overweight and suffer from countless symptoms that this stage of life can bring. Often, I see the pattern occurring where women feed each other with negativity, creating even more anxiety and low mood.

I can assure you that it is entirely possible to boost your mood and help you feel more in control of your body and mind by learning to become more positive. Of course, this takes time and you need to expect results to come to you cumulatively and not overnight. Whilst positivity will not automatically remove your troubles and worries, it will allow you to cope with them in much healthier and more productive ways. You will start to see challenges as learning curves, rather than instantly being laid low by them. This can be extremely useful during the menopause, when challenges may come your way on a regular basis.

There are many ways to practice positivity and I want to mention two techniques, that are particularly useful for helping you to see the glass as half full instead of half empty. They are called positive affirmation and reframing. Applying these two methods will have far-reaching benefits on your life as they will open your mind to the opportunities around you, and who knows where they may lead?

Method Number One – Positive Affirmations

Affirmations are positive statements that you keep repeating to yourself. It is a powerful activity which can help you change the way you think and remove negative language that you have a habit of using when talking to yourself. This technique can help you to become more positive and overcome your negative thinking and behaviours. It has been proven that the repetition of statements can positively affect your conscious and unconscious mind.

Here are 15 affirmations that can change your state of mind and help you stay positive. Repeat them out loud several times a day and focus on their meaning. Early morning and before bedtime are two the best times for this. At first you might find it a little strange, but the more you do it, the more you will feel confident doing it. Watch your thoughts during this activity, believe your words, and they will become real.

- I am strong

- I am positive

- I am unique

- I am powerful

- I am fearless

- I am attractive

- I am confident

- I am smart

- I love my body

- I fully accept myself

- I am proud of myself

- I truly love myself

- I am grateful for everything I have

- I am who I want to be

- I am enough

Method Number Two – Reframing

Another powerful method for practising positivity is called reframing. It is a type of cognitive behavioural therapy technique that replaces a negative thought with a positive one. This technique helps you to become more aware of your self-talk and the effects it has on you.

Here is how it might work in practice:

- You have a negative thought and you acknowledge it as negative, e.g. "I have lines under my eyes, and I hate them".

- You take this negative thought and turn it into something positive, e.g. "I have lines under my eyes, which show my wisdom and experience".

- You would then repeat this new thought several times, and every time you notice the lines under your eyes you would repeat it again.

- Repetition is critical here because, over time, your brain will think of the positive thought, before the negative one and assume that to be true.

The more you reframe negative thoughts that pop into your mind, the more you will become a generally more positive person overall.

A combination of doing positive affirmation and practising reframing can significantly impact the way you feel about yourself and the direction your life is going to take.

Give it a try! It is very easy to apply them in your everyday life. They will enhance your life not just in overcoming the negative mental health effects of the menopause but also helping you be a more positive person. This will improve your relationship with others and help you to be much kinder to yourself.

Meditation and Mindfulness

Many women find that practising mindfulness can help them to feel happier and more uplifted. Adopting mindfulness in your life will allow you to be present and live in the moment, rather than thinking about the past, or jumping ahead and worrying about the future.

If you find meditation difficult at first, persevere. It is hard to quieten your mind when you have been so used to all the noise around you, but you can develop it with time. Mindfulness meditation is often easier than regular meditation because you can do it on the go. All you need to do is be aware of what is around you. So, the next time you are out walking, avoid looking at your phone and instead tune into your surroundings.

First, calm your mind by focusing on your breathing. Notice the inhaling and exhaling, and keep it controlled and slow. When you are ready, start to observe your surroundings; look at the leaves and how they shine in the light, watch the playful dog running in the field, and see how the clouds move slowly in the sky. The more tuned you are to the present, the more you will be able to simply observe your troubles rather than feel like you need to do something about them, e.g. react emotionally. As thoughts enter your mind, simply acknowledge them but do not overthink it; allow them to float back out and return at a later time, when you are more concerned with them.

With practice, this all becomes much easier.

Just as being positive can help you live in a more upbeat and happier way, mindfulness can help you deal with upheaval more effectively and improve your mood. You will start to see the menopause as something that is simply happening to you, not as something which defines you or changes your future. As a result, you will not obsess or worry over small changes, and you will not allow your confidence to be ruined.

Rest When You Need to

A lot is going on inside your body right now and this means you might feel tired from time to time or even experience fatigue. This is a common complaint from menopausal women, and it is further compounded if you are already struggling to get a good night's sleep.

If you are suffering from fatigue, be kind to yourself and rest whenever you need to. Give yourself permission to listen to your body and make sure you slow down. We all need a little downtime; in fact, it should be on prescription!

Far too many women feel like they have to take on the world and win every single time, but this is an unrealistic expectation and it is not healthy either. Putting too much expectation on yourself will lead to burn out.

Take the time to slow down and focus on doing what your body is asking you to do. You are not failing, you are simply doing what your body needs. As Jim Rohn said "Take care of your body. It is the only place you have to live".

At the moment, your body is dealing with changes and your hormones are fluctuating, some days you might need more rest than others. Simply monitor how you feel on a daily basis and change your routine accordingly. If you feel like everything is on top of you and there is a to-do list as long as your arm to complete, work through it slowly and methodically. Similarly, if you feel you need to take a moment, take it. Listen to your body and let "how you feel" be your guide.

Regular Exercise

There are several chemicals released in the body during exercise. Some of these are dopamine, serotonin and endorphins. They are brain chemicals that create happy feelings and are known to lift the mood. Exercise can help you feel more upbeat and positive, and as you already learnt, it can be great for controlling hot flushes too. As you can see, there are many benefits from just getting your body moving a little bit more. And if you can incorporate outdoor exercise with fresh air at the same time, you will notice even more benefits.

The healing effects of Mother Nature are ideal for helping to banish worries and relieve stress.

If you have a friend who also wants to exercise more, why not head out together? You will get a social boost, and you will be exercising at the same time.

Eat Nourishing, Healthy Foods

Eating a healthy diet is beneficial on many different levels, but certain foods can give you the feel-good factor and boost your mood, while others you should try and avoid. You might love a glass of wine in the evening, but you need to proceed with caution. Alcohol is a depressant, and more than one glass could easily tip you towards the lower end of the scale.

Reducing caffeine intake would also be beneficial, as caffeine is a stimulant that can cause anxiety for anyone prone to it.

Here is what you should eat to boost your mood:

- Fatty types of fish, full of healthy omega-3 fatty acids, such as sardines, mackerel, etc.

- Dark chocolate – in moderation!

- Bananas

- Oats

- Fermented foods such as kefir and sauerkraut

- Berries

- Nuts

- Seeds

These super healthy foods are known to help with depression, stabilise your blood sugar levels and improve your mood, and increase feel-good chemicals in your brain and your gut. You can easily incorporate them into your diet. Try to experiment with different recipes and learn new and exciting ways to prepare your meals. It is far easier than you think to pack several healthy ingredients into one meal; you simply need to think creatively and be mindful of what you need in your daily diet.

I strongly suggest you cook your meals rather than relying on fast-food and processed foods. Processed foods will not help your menopausal symptoms. In fact, they are widely known to encourage your symptoms to get much worse.

Some of my clients find it very therapeutic to cook their meals from scratch. It is about being creative and making something from basics with their hands. Creativity and cooking together are known to boost the feel-good factor and help with improving your mood. When you add in the ingredients that are also linked to mood improvement, you are onto a good thing.

One of my clients did exactly that – she started experimenting with new recipes and cooking meals from scratch using fresh ingredients.

She was very obese and unhealthy when we began working together. She felt uncomfortable about her physical appearance and was struggling with her self-worth. Then, everything changed!

She started cooking healthy recipes with her two daughters. Spending time with them and cooking healthy meals twice a week brought so much enjoyment to her. The whole family benefited from this experience. My client developed a much closer relationship with her teenage daughters. Also, enjoying healthy foods and eating meals together had a positive effect on the health of the whole family.

If you have not already downloaded a *Healthy Eating for Menopause – Recipe Book*, please visit <u>bit.ly/menopause-</u>

healthy-recipes-2 and download your free copy. You will find plenty of delicious recipes there.

Try Yoga

Yoga teaches you to control your breathing and use it as a grounding tool. Whenever you are feeling stressed, tired, or upset, you can go back to your breathing and slow things down. This is a very calming and healthy way to control stress and anxiety. Yoga has been shown to improve mood, but it could also help strengthen the body and reduce the chances of muscle loss, which could lead to osteoporosis in later life. By incorporating yoga into your daily life, you are giving yourself a tool you can use whenever you feel stressed, upset, angry, tired, or experience any other negative emotion.

Yoga does not have to be about being super-flexible, and there are many different positions you can try that allow you to start from the bottom and work your way up. If you have any problems with your back or another part of the body, you can simply tell the instructor and they will show you a way to perform the yoga pose without aggravating your pre-existing problem.

Allow Yourself a Social Life

At the end of a long working day, you might feel like hiding away, and when you are feeling a little low in mood, that is most probably what you feel like doing. However, hiding away is not going to make you feel better, and it is likely to further worsen your low mood and anxiety.

There is strength in friendship and even if you are just going to your friend's house for a cup of tea, or you are going out for a meal, make sure you create time for a social life. This is not being indulgent, and it is not a waste of money; it is a vital part of your overall health and well-being and as far as your mental health is concerned, it is crucial. However, there are limits and if you are always out drinking and partying, or maybe you are heading out for food a lot, you might want to rein things in a little and question why you are spending all your spare time and attention in that direction. Remember, everything in moderation.

Find Support from Other Women

A great way to feel stronger within yourself is to surround yourself with equally strong women who are going through the same thing as you. Check online, find local support groups for menopausal women, or ask your doctor for information on community groups you could join. You could even look on social media and find Facebook support groups that suit your needs.

Fear of the unknown, not understanding what is happening to you, or feeling like no-one else is going through the same thing can usually worsen low mood and anxiety. Surround yourself with other women who are in the same situation can help you feel stronger, more confident, and ultimately, more positive within yourself.

Seek Help if You Need It

The self-help methods that I mentioned will help you to feel more upbeat and help you be more in control of your mood and any anxiety you may experience. However, there is a fine line between feeling low and being depressed. It is vital to recognise this as struggling with low mood for too long can lead to depression.

For many people, admitting they are feeling depressed, anxious, agitated, etc. can be a huge uphill battle, but you must take that first step. Visit your doctor and be open about how you are feeling. You do not have to struggle and there are many treatment options your doctor may be able to explore with you in order to find the one that suits you best. Seeing a counsellor and receiving help with your feelings is worth considering. Or HRT could be the right option for you. It can help with mood-related menopausal symptoms. But there are also other options available that you can explore with your doctor.

Simply know that help is there if you need it. You do not have to struggle your way through the menopause feeling less than yourself. Mental health is something we all need to learn to take just as seriously as our physical health.

Key Points

- The menopause can cause mood swings, agitation, stress, anxiety and low confidence.

- Problems with mental health as a result of the menopause should not be ignored, and you should seek help from your doctor if you find these symptoms particularly troublesome.

- You can use several self-help methods to boost your mood, including exercising regularly, changing your diet, trying mindfulness with yoga, and others.

- HRT may be offered to you if you are struggling with mood during the menopause, but you do not have to take if you do not want to. I suggest that you talk to your doctor about alternatives.

- Always reach out for help if you are struggling with your mental health. You can seek support from family, friends, and other women who are going through the same thing as you.

Chapter 6

Where Has Your Desire Gone?

With hormones causing all manner of confusion and upset within your body during the perimenopause and menopause, it is hardly surprising that sex is likely to be the last thing on your mind.

During the menopause, many women experience decreased desire, however it is equally as possible that your libido will shoot through the roof and your experience will be very different. Again, you have hormones to thank for all of this, but understanding how you can deal with a loss of libido in particular is a vital part of overcoming the struggles of the menopause.

You might think that lacking sex drive is not a big deal in the grand scheme of things, and for some women it probably is not, but if your partner's needs and expectations are different, then it can be quite difficult for both of you to deal with it. As a result, you might experience problems within your relationship and start noticing that your confidence drops. Many women feel more confident when they are having regular sex with their partner, and losing the desire for it or experiencing vaginal dryness, can drastically affect the way they feel about themselves.

There are several difficulties with the loss of libido. Firstly, some women can be very sexually active, but they begin to notice changes occurring in this department when they approach the menopause. You might start to feel confused as to why you are not feeling the desire as much anymore, or in some cases not at all. This could take your confidence away or even make you feel unattractive.

Secondly, you might start experiencing relationship issues because of this. Your partner needs to understand very clearly why you are feeling this way, which requires you to have open and honest communication with each other. Otherwise, your partner might conclude that you are not sexually attracted to them anymore. In some cases, that can cause serious issues within a relationship.

I believe that sexual intimacy between couples is important for maintaining a connection and keeping the desire alive, and if you fail to talk to your partner and let them know what is going on, it could be damaging for your relationship. Therefore, it is crucial that you open up and perhaps let your partner help you too; your partner may turn out to be your main ally against the menopause if you share your problems with them.

Of course, we have already explored the fact that hormonal imbalances cause your loss of libido, with dwindling testosterone levels being the main culprit. If you want to, you can take testosterone supplements, but these do come with their fair share of side effects, which may not be very beneficial when you weigh up the pros versus the cons. If you want to explore this possibility, consulting your doctor might be a good idea, and make sure to listen to both sides of the argument before making a final decision.

Why is Libido Affected During the Menopause?

For some women, being menopausal simply means having no interest in sex. We know about the hormonal side of things, but what else can cause loss of libido during the menopause? It is not all about oestrogen, progesterone and testosterone for once. There are also a few other issues leading to these menopausal symptoms.

I have already mentioned the fact that during the menopause many women put on weight and find it harder to lose. Any excess weight can change the way you feel about yourself and affect your body confidence. Feeling this way might prevent you from being intimate with your partner and also stop you from enjoying sex.

Another common reason for the loss of libido with menopausal women is caused by the symptoms which they experience. Menopausal symptoms can make you feel generally uncomfortable, e.g. hot flushes, night sweats, and feeling tired in general. These can drastically reduce your desire to have sex.

Another symptom that is sex-related is vaginal dryness. These two symptoms are often interlinked and can cause upheaval in your relationship, and can drastically affect your confidence, if you allow them to.

Other reasons, such as feeling low in mood, anxious, or depressed, will undoubtedly affect your sexual desire. Suffering from depression can cause a lack of interest in sex, and it is usually one of the first symptoms that people notice. It is not surprising that women going through the menopause will not feel like having sex when their mood is affected.

Sex is supposed to be enjoyable, something that brings you closer to your partner. Therefore, it is understandable why both parties might feel unhappy with the situation you find yourself in, and frustrated about the issues you are experiencing.

If your lack of libido prevents you from enjoying this part of your relationship with your partner, it is important not to feel guilty about how this affects both of your lives. Both you and your partner must understand that this is not something you are choosing not to do, therefore communicating with each other during this time is vital.

Showing understanding towards each other's needs will strengthen your relationship and help you explore how to be intimate and close in other ways. Communicating your worries with your partner and respecting each other's wishes is vital at any stage of your relationship.

Can You Boost Your Libido?

As I have already mentioned, a reduced sex drive can create problems in the relationship and talking to your partner about it is important. Being honest about how you are feeling can help you explore your relationship intimacy and find different ways to be close to each other.

271

However, we will cover relationship issues later in this chapter.

There are some ways you can try and boost your libido, and get yourself in the mood if you do miss a little heat.

Discuss HRT or Testosterone with Your Doctor

HRT might be able to help you with low libido and it could be an option for you if you choose to take it. As discussed previously, it can help with other menopausal symptoms too.

Throughout your life, your testosterone levels gradually decline and this can have a tremendous effect on your sex drive. There are also other benefits of testosterone such as maintaining muscle and bone strength and having normal cognitive functioning. If HRT is not helping you, then taking testosterone supplements could be another option for you. The issue with testosterone, however, is that it can, in some cases, cause excessive hair growth and acne for some women. It is important to be aware of this side effect before you decide to take it.

Try Lubricants

Some women use lubricants to make the whole process easier. This ensures sex is more comfortable and enjoyable. Many couples choose to use lubricants as part of their sex life regardless, so definitely give it a try.

Regular Exercise

Exercise is recommended for every menopausal side effect. It is an almost magical solution! Regular exercise releases those feel-good endorphins which can trigger sexual arousal and boost circulation which is useful for women who are trying to feel more in the mood.

Exercising will make you feel better in yourself and that could be enough to enhance your desire.

Try Kegel Exercises

Kegel exercises are commonly used to strengthen the pelvic floor, especially during aging and after pregnancy, but it can be used for other reasons too. When you regularly do Kegel exercises you are boosting the circulation, which can make sex more enjoyable.

If you have never done Kegel exercises before, try this:

- First, you need to find the pelvic floor muscles to contract in the first place. When you urinate, you would contract your pelvic floor to stop the stream. That is the muscle you are looking for.

- Once you have figured out the right muscle, squeeze it for five seconds, counting slowly and steadily.

- Release the squeeze as you slowly and steadily count to five again.

- The ideal amount of exercises to do is 10 repetitions and you should try and do them three times per day. You might have to build up slowly, but that should be your aim.

Regularly practising Kegel exercises will help the blood flow, lubrication and sensitivity of the vagina which will make sex much more enjoyable.

Cognitive Behavioural Therapy (CBT)

A possible treatment method for women who feel distressed from their low libido is to try CBT. It is a form of mindset training therapy used for a wide range of different problems and conditions. It can help you deal with the menopause symptoms that relate to your mood, and if your libido is affected directly because of that, you might find this therapy very helpful.

During the menopause and especially during the postmenopausal period it is very common to experience vaginal dryness. It causes discomfort and can make intercourse extremely uncomfortable and even painful. When you combine the possibility of vaginal dryness with the chance of a reduced libido, you can see why menopausal women are struggling with the idea of sex during this time of life. Sex is supposed to be fun, intimate and carefree — yet many women struggle with pain and discomfort.

In the next section, we will explore why vaginal dryness can be a problem for women, debunk your worries about whether it is dangerous or not, and figure out how to manage the problem overall.

How to Overcome Vaginal Dryness

You have learnt so far that low levels of oestrogen and progesterone are responsible for most of the problems that occur during the menopause, and it is certainly the cause for vaginal dryness.

Some women only notice vaginal dryness as a problem during sexual intercourse, but others notice it more regularly. It can even happen while walking or wearing tight clothes. This is a massive problem for some postmenopausal women when oestrogen and progesterone are at an all-time low. As a result, the vagina is dry, and there is a risk of developing a condition called atrophic vaginitis or atrophy.

The medical name does sound scary, but it is a very common condition that affects many women; some women have this and are not even aware of it. Atrophic vaginitis or vaginal atrophy is when the vagina's tissues are not being nourished by oestrogen and progesterone, and as a result, they can become thinner. Simply wearing tight underwear can cause irritation and pain, sometimes resulting in bleeding. Of course, any bleeding after the menopause should be investigated by your doctor, and irritated vaginal atrophy or vaginitis can often be the cause of it.

Vaginal dryness is not dangerous per se, and the conditions associated with it will not cause you any real harm, but it is an uncomfortable and sometimes extremely painful condition to have. Thankfully it is possible to sort it out quite easily, and it is something we will explore next. I will give you some suggestions on what you can do to resolve it, so that your quality of life is not affected by this problem.

- *Have sex* – Regular sex has been shown to keep vaginal tissues healthy and help to reduce vaginal dryness and the possibility of atrophy after the menopause. It is quite ironic that loss of libido is one of the main symptoms of the menopause and even after the menopause, and as a result you might not feel like helping yourself to one of the best routes towards less vaginal dryness.

- *Use vaginal moisturisers regularly* – Using vaginal moisturisers every few days can reduce vaginal dryness and defend against the possibility of atrophy. Look for brands such as KY Jelly or Replens.

- *Use lubricants during sex* – Applying a few drops of lubricant just before sex can help to make the whole thing more comfortable and therefore more enjoyable for you and your partner. This will also help reduce pain and, as a result, you are more likely to relax and not always anticipate a painful reaction. Women who experience a large degree of vaginal dryness can lead to another potential problem called dyspareunia. It is persistent pain which usually occurs during sex, but can also happen before and after. In some cases, this can be very painful and can ruin a woman's sex life, but treatment is about learning to relax and allowing the vaginal muscles to do the same. Sexual responses are just as psychological as they are physiological, so be sure to focus on relaxation and take your time, if this is a problem for you.

- *Vaginal oestrogen* – Your doctor may prescribe you vaginal oestrogen at a low dose, which you can apply either as a cream, take as a tablet, or insert in a ring form. This approach helps to nourish the vaginal tissues and puts back some of the oestrogen you lack, due to the menopause. This will help to avoid vaginal atrophy and reduce the problem. However, vaginal oestrogen is not for everyone and if you have had breast cancer in the past or have a strong family history of it, you will need to discuss this carefully with your doctor to weigh up the pros and cons versus the risks.

- *Vaginal suppository (dehydroepiandrosterone)* – Your doctor might suggest a vaginal suppository that you insert every night, containing DHEA or Dehydroepiandrosterone. This can help if you are suffering from painful intercourse as a result of vaginal dryness. A suppository such as this will help to nourish the tissues and help you relax as a result.

- *Ospemifene tablets* – This medication helps with painful intercourse caused by vaginal atrophy and dryness, but if you or anyone in your family has had breast cancer, this solution is not suitable for you.

In conclusion, I just want to say that if you are suffering from vagina dryness and it is affecting your life, you do not have to face it without help; it is simply a case of finding the right route forwards for your situation. There are many ways you can help to nourish your vaginal area and make everything less painful and more comfortable, whether you are attempting to have sex or not.

If this is a big problem for you, be sure to speak to your doctor as there are some prescription treatments you can try for severe cases. This is especially relevant if you notice dryness and discomfort during the day, when walking, sitting, or when wearing particular types of clothes.

Talk to Your Partner

If you are in a relationship, it is vital that you are open and honest about your feelings with your partner and that you have honest communication with each other. Your partner may not understand the symptoms of the menopause and what is happening inside your body. Therefore, communicating your issues, worries, and desires is the key.

Whilst you should certainly never feel guilty for your libido problem, you also need to understand how the situation can impact upon your partner. Being honest and communicating openly is vital. It would be best if you talked to your partner to get them to understand and be sympathetic towards your situation.

By becoming emotionally closer to your partner in this way, you might also notice that your libido starts to come back a little. There are other ways to be intimate with your partner without having sexual intercourse, so spend time together, make date nights a priority, go back to holding hands, kissing, and caressing each other, and these forms of intimacy might help to boost your libido. If nothing else, they will bring you closer together as a couple and that could give you the extra boost of support you need to overcome the challenges you are facing in the menopause.

In some cases, sex drive can be a little like a muscle you work out at the gym. The more you work on it, the stronger it becomes. So, if your lack of or lower libido is a problem for you, work on making it stronger via non-sexual intimacy and see if it starts to trickle back into your life slowly. Many women find that it does.

However, after all this discussion about low libido, perhaps you are one of the women who notice a higher sex drive during the menopause! In that case, it could be a good thing or a bad thing for you; however, your partner is likely to find it a fantastic new development!

Key Points

- Loss of libido is very common during the menopause and can also be connected to weight gain, loss of confidence or low mood.

- You must communicate with your partner to ensure that relationship problems do not occur due to a lack of sexual intimacy.

- There are a few ways to increase libido, including considering HRT or testosterone treatment, lubricants, CBT and regular exercise.

- Vaginal dryness is a common side effect of the menopause caused by reduced sex hormones, and it can contribute to loss of libido due to uncomfortable intercourse.

- Using vaginal moisturisers and lubricants are the most common ways to overcome vaginal dryness.

- Work on becoming emotionally closer to your partner during this time to maintain or even to improve your relationship.

Chapter 7

The Importance of Avoiding Toxins

As if we do not have enough to deal with during the menopause, it is important to be aware of outside influences that may cause more problems.

In this case, I am talking about toxins in general healthcare products.

Did you know that anything from shampoo to body lotion, and makeup remover to moisturiser can contain chemicals which can play havoc with your hormones? Also, pesticides and other harmful substances are used during the manufacturing process of certain fresh produce, which can also affect your hormones.

During the menopause you have enough going on, there is plenty to throw your hormonal balance out of sync as it is, so being aware of the toxins that can add to your troubles is vital. You can then work to decrease them and possibly even reduce your symptoms considerably.

In this chapter, we will look at why some toxins can affect your hormones, the ones you should try and avoid, and how you can find alternatives, so you are not missing out on any of your favourite health and beauty products.

Why Are Toxins Troublesome During the Menopause?

Certain products contain chemical-based ingredients to prolong their shelf life, add attractive colours to their appearance, or boost the effectiveness of a natural ingredient. On the whole, many of these ingredients are considered "safe", although only in small amounts. What that "safe" label does not take into account is the effect that the ongoing use can have on the body and how it affects your endocrine system.

We already know that the endocrine system is responsible for many of your body's hormones. This can affect the big three hormones, which are affected during the menopause too — oestrogen, progesterone, and testosterone. By using products with a high amount of chemicals or toxins, you are certainly adding fuel to the fire.

Your hormones are already out of balance naturally at this stage of your life, but by continuing to use products that include toxins, you are increasing the detrimental effects, and therefore worsening your menopausal symptoms. The worst aspect of it all is that many women have no idea that their health and beauty products may have this effect on their symptoms, and they continue using them without even realising the dangers.

Some of the most common toxins which you need to avoid are parabens, ureas and sulphate. In the next section I will give you a comprehensive list, but you have no doubt heard of at least two of them.

Whilst the health and beauty industry has made a concerted effort to reduce the amount of toxins in their products, simply because the ingredients list of products are now subject to more scrutiny than ever before, they are still in there albeit in smaller amounts. By cutting these harmful chemicals out completely, you could help to reduce your hot flushes, night sweats, and other troublesome symptoms, simply by changing your beauty routine a little.

These toxins are known as "endocrine disrupting chemicals", and this means that they cause your hormones to be completely deranged. That is not what you need right now!

Your body cannot tell the difference between many of these toxins (which mimic the effects of oestrogen) and natural oestrogen, which can cause extra stress within your body and increase the number of menopausal symptoms you are experiencing, linked to your hormones. Besides, they can damage your insulin-producing cells, disrupt the hormones released from your thyroid gland, and cause your body's natural detoxing system to be completely out of sync.

Hormones are very closely linked. It is common for women to gain weight during the menopause because the distortion in oestrogen and progesterone also affects ghrelin and leptin, which tells you when you are full or hungry.

I have already mentioned the fact that thyroid hormones can be disrupted due to the imbalance of oestrogen. All hormones affect one another in some way, so when toxins affect one hormone, you can expect a knock-on effect with the others, particularly when it comes to oestrogen imbalance.

Hidden Toxins in Personal Care Products

Most health and beauty products are applied to the skin and absorbed. If products contain these toxins, or fake/synthetic oestrogen (more on that shortly), they are absorbed into the blood stream and cause your existing imbalance to deteriorate.

Let's look at some of the most common toxins you need to try and cut out of your health and beauty routine. You can learn what is in each of your favourite products by simply reading the ingredients on the back — manufacturers now have to mention if they include any of these toxins, so it is worthwhile becoming better informed about the contents of the products you use.

- **BPA** – This is a chemical which is regularly used in plastic products, but it is used in some health and beauty products, packaged to actually imitate oestrogen, thereby acting as a synthetic, or fake, oestrogen. BPAs have links with various types of cancer, reproductive issues, heart disease, and early cases of puberty.

- **Dioxin** – Dioxin is used in many different products and packaging types. Dioxin is famous for disrupting sex hormones and can stay in the body for quite a long time. It is also very hard to avoid, so you need to become alert and cautious when reading packaging before using products.

- *Atrazine* – Studies with atrazine have found that it interacts with sex hormones. Again, we are looking at a further disruption to oestrogen here. Atrazine also has a link with breast tumors and puberty delays, amongst many other general health issues.

- *Phthalates* – There are many studies which link phthalates to hormonal changes and problems with the thyroid gland. Phthalates also affect the male reproductive system but have been shown to cause havoc with hormones in general.

- *Parabens* – More and more health and beauty products are trying to cut out parabens in their products, but this is a work in progress for many. Parabens imitate oestrogen and is likely to cause your current menopausal symptoms to change or worsen, due to a further imbalance. Parabens have also been shown to cause problems with other hormones whilst also affecting the reproductive system.

- *Sulphates* – A little like parabens, sulphates can be found in many health and beauty products, although there is a concerted effort to try and reduce this. Sulphates act as synthetic oestrogen, thereby causing many menopausal symptoms to worsen, whilst also increasing the risk of disruption to thyroid hormones.

It is not only health and beauty products you need to be careful of. Many chemicals and toxins can be found in various foods, generally originating from how they are grown or manufactured. There is a concerted push to reduce manufacturing that includes fake hormones or pesticides, but they continue to occur.

If you can, I suggest that you shop organically. Yes, these products can cost a little more, but they are a much healthier alternative to conventionally grown produce. They contain a higher level of antioxidants and have far less synthetic chemicals.

Eating organic foods will help you avoid the likelihood of ingesting pesticides and other manufacturing toxins. Clean eating helps menopausal women to manage their symptoms better.

Buying a filter for your water is a wise investment. There are many contaminants found in drinking water and even though this is classed as safe to drink, it may contain traces of toxins that could affect your hormones. If you drink filtered water only, you will avoid this risk, and you will be drinking cleaner and healthier water as a result.

Alternative Products to Try

First things first, not all health and beauty products contain toxins, and you should become used to reading labels and knowing what to look for. In addition to the toxins mentioned earlier, you should also avoid any product which lists the following ingredients on their packaging:

- Fragrance

- Artificial colours

- Petroleum

- Formaldehyde

- Preservatives

- Foaming agents

- Antibacterial agents

- Plasticisers

- Siloxanes

- PEG compounds

The best suggestion I can give you is to cut out some of the products which you know contain toxins and see how you feel after a week or two. If you notice a difference in your menopausal symptoms or you simply feel better in yourself, try and find an alternative to that particular product. It is not always easy to pinpoint one specific product, especially if you have a bathroom cabinet brimming with different lotions, potions, and creams! By swapping some of the products you use most often, perhaps one by one, you will be able to identify which is causing you the biggest issue.

Try looking for products that contain organic or natural ingredients only. These will be marked as such, but again, read the labels to be sure. You might also like to try making your own products in some cases, such as body scrubs, exfoliators, moisturisers, etc. You might not be able to do this with all your favourite health and beauty products, but if you check online you will find a range of "recipes" to make completely natural products. This can also be quite fun, and you could gift these to friends too.

Avoiding toxins can not only help you with your menopausal symptoms but can lead to better overall health and well-being and reduce risk factors for developing chronic or severe diseases.

Key Points

This chapter has covered the importance of understanding how toxins and chemicals contained within health and beauty products may affect your hormones. You might not have even been aware of this before, but you may have heard about a few of the ingredients mentioned in this book.

By reducing your exposure to toxins, you may find that your menopausal symptoms reduce or even themselves out a little. Of course, this also reduces your risk of developing serious health problems as a result of too much exposure over time.

The main points to remember from this chapter are:

- Certain toxins found in health and beauty products can mimic the effects of oestrogen, as well as progesterone and testosterone. The body does not know how to differentiate between natural and synthetic oestrogen, therefore these products add to your menopausal problems.

- Manufacturers are now required to list all ingredients on their packaging, so in order to avoid your exposure to common toxins, always read labels thoroughly.

- Parabens, sulphates and BPA are three of the most common types of toxins that affect hormones, however, there is a long list of the most dangerous types to avoid.

- Look for products that are labelled as organic or natural.

- Shop for organic produce to avoid your exposure to dangerous pesticides, and other toxins used in the manufacturing process.

- Use a water filter to cut out any contaminants in your water.

- Try cutting out products one by one and seeing how you feel in yourself; this will show you if one particular product and its associated toxins are affecting your hormones or not.

Chapter 8

Palpitations and Headaches, What is The Deal?

The menopause can throw some very odd symptoms at you and two of the most difficult to deal with are palpitations and headaches. They occur in two very different parts of the body, but they can be related or unrelated, and can be part of your menopausal journey.

Why does the menopause cause these particular symptoms?

In the earlier chapters, I blamed hormones for almost everything that happens to us, and they definitely cause these occasional headaches and palpitations.

The reason for this is because of the changing levels of hormones in your body. It is common for palpitations to occur during hot flushes as you notice your heart beating a little faster. And for women who experience hormone-related headaches that often occur during or before their monthly cycle, they could start having severe and frequent headaches.

Palpitations usually disappear as quickly as they appear, but they can be upsetting whilst they are there. If you notice you are suffering from palpitations, sit down, breathe steadily and wait for it to pass. It is important to remain calm and remember that nothing is going to hurt you; most of the time palpitations are harmless.

In this chapter, I am going to focus on these two troubling symptoms and give you some advice on how to reduce them.

Some women may go through the menopause and never notice even one palpitation, whilst some may have lots of them. Some women may go through the menopause and not have more headaches than they usually would have. Some women have them regularly. It is a personalised deal and it is important to know what your version of normal is.

The Importance of Monitoring Palpitations and Headaches

Whilst both palpitations and headaches are not harmful in general, they can occur due to underlying causes in some situations. That means it is vital that you monitor them and get anything checked out that does not feel right to you. This advice is the same for all other symptoms I have mentioned in this book.

If you notice that you are getting more headaches and palpitations, it is good to keep a symptom diary. This will give your doctor more information to work with, and they will be able to understand whether there is a pattern to your symptoms. This will help your doctor to diagnose your problem more easily.

In rare cases, both palpitations and headaches can be due to more sinister reasons, but these are few and far between, and both symptoms are very common in regular life. In fact, both can be caused by stress, which we are going to cover in more detail next.

The Link with Stress and How to Reduce It

Stress can cause all manner of symptoms to occur within the body and most of the time you do not even know you are stressed!

We live in stressful times and that means that most of us are operating within a constantly heightened state of awareness. The body has its own stress response, more commonly known as the "fight or flight" response.

When your brain observes something and thinks of it as a threat, it gives your body everything it needs to either fight the danger, or run away from it. The problem is that your brain will always remember negative past experiences and perceive new situations as a threat. This might make you feel constantly stressed out and result in increased cortisol levels. Cortisol is the stress hormone, contributing to the imbalance of hormones you already have due to the menopause.

Stress can cause headaches and it can also cause heart palpitations. When stress is prolonged, the body does not know how to differentiate between a normal state and a stressed state. As a result, regular uncomfortable symptoms occur, such as trouble sleeping, appetite problems (eating too little or too much), low mood, agitation and headaches.

The good news is that you have more control than you realise. Stress might seem like it is controlling your life, but you can change your lifestyle and take back control of your own ship.

It might take a little time, but little by little you will notice that you feel better in yourself. There are no downsides to focusing on stress reduction, so make this your aim whether you are suffering from palpitations and headaches or not.

In today's society, we are constantly subjected to stress. It is such a chronic state of being, that we might not even be aware of all the ways in which we might be experiencing stress. In order to manage your stress effectively it is important to find out what is causing it. Identifying your stressors is the first step towards having a stress-free life.

The following exercise can help you to recognise your stressors and find different ways of removing them from your life. Follow these five simple steps:

1. Take a piece of paper or a notebook and brainstorm your stressors – It might be something that is massive, or it might be very small. If it is

affecting your stress levels, it is important. Never pass something off as too small; if it is bothering you, it is large enough to take notice of.

2. Write them down.

3. Is there one thing you can pinpoint, or are there several?

4. Work out how you can address those problems. Remember, some of them you may not be able to address immediately.

5. Draw a plan to overcome your stressors. Use the piece of paper or write it in your notebook. Working out a plan puts you in charge and creates a feeling of being in control of your life. It is a great confidence boost and an excellent motivational tool.

I hope that this exercise will help you to identify your stressors, so you can make changes that will help you reduce your stress levels.

Sitting down and doing some soul searching might not be enough for some people. If this is the case, I suggest you follow the rules for stress management. Most common tips include:

- Exercise regularly

- Reduce your caffeine and alcohol intake

- Reduce how much sugar you eat

- Do your best to get a good night's sleep

- Meditate and practice mindfulness

- Be positive

Stress is not something you should be inviting into your life, and learning how to reduce the amount of stress you are experiencing is vital for your health and happiness too. Of course, this will also help to reduce any troubling symptoms you are experiencing, including previously mentioned headaches and palpitations.

Anxiety is another symptom of the menopause and it has a strong link with stress.

It has been shown that stress aggravates the symptoms of anxiety. Therefore, you must learn the cause of your anxiety and understand its connection with stress.

Some people feel shaky or distant when their anxiety is spiking, whilst others feel heavy and hot. Learn to recognise your feelings of anxiety, as this will help you to intervene if things start to deteriorate. Getting familiar with your triggers will help you to manage them better and reduce the severity they might have on your life. Many women learn to do this before the menopause, such is the prevalence of anxiety in modern society.

The constant attack of stress can lead to hormonal disorders like adrenal fatigue, in which your adrenal glands (responsible for producing your stress hormones) become overworked and begin to wear out. This leads to physical fatigue, lack of motivation and depression.

Metabolic disorders are hormonal as well, and conditions like insulin or leptin resistance can cause an increase in your stress hormones, which create a downward spiral of hormonal dysfunction.

Hormonal health is particularly fragile in menopausal women as their bodies naturally start to alter the production of hormones. This is perfectly normal and natural, but it does cause a shift in the entire endocrine system. By introducing outside factors to the mix, like diet and environment, this change then becomes exponentially more difficult for the body to adjust to.

Natural Methods to Reduce Palpitations and Headaches

Palpitations and headaches might not be the worst of your menopausal problems. Perhaps you suffer from hot flushes far more than headaches, and maybe you do not have palpitations at all. However, you might be plagued with them. In either situation, knowing what to do to reduce them naturally is a good thing.

I am aware that today many people reach for painkillers even when they feel the slightest pain somewhere in the body. I understand that sometimes it is necessary to take them in order to numb the pain, but I am not a fan of taking them regularly.

There are countless reasons why you might be experiencing heart palpitations or headaches. It could be because of some underlying condition that you have, or changes in your hormone levels, or due to stress.

Here, I would like to highlight natural processes to deal with the issues of palpitations and headaches.

Natural Methods to Reduce Palpitations:

- *Regularly use relaxation techniques* – Deep breathing, exercise, and meditation are ideal ways to relax your mind and body and reduce palpitations. When you are experiencing a palpitation, try to focus on your breathing and slow it down. As a result, the palpitation will pass much faster and you will not become anxious or worried about the feeling. Remember, palpitations can last for a second or a few minutes, but they are not dangerous, so do not be too worried about them. You should also try practising relaxation in general, as this will help you get a good night's sleep, something that can be difficult for some menopausal women to achieve.

- *Cut down on stimulants* – Try to do your best to cut down on stimulants. Consuming stimulants such as caffeine, tobacco, alcohol and sugar are bad habits that could be extremely damaging to your health, and are also known to increase the risk of palpitations. Remember that caffeine can also be in other drinks aside from coffee, such as cola, tea, and even in chocolate. If you can cut down on the amount of sugar you consume, that will positively affect your hot flushes and the number of palpitations you have.

- ***Work on your vagus nerve*** – The vagus nerve carries signals between your brain and throughout the rest of your body. By stimulating your vagus nerve, you can learn to reduce the number of palpitations you experience as you can slow down your heart rate to a steady and regular rhythm. This may not mean that palpitations are never experienced, but they should be far less frequent. A few ways to do this include:

  o Exposure to cold temperatures (do this with caution, however, as too much cold too quickly can cause shock – a cold compress is enough)

  o Breathing deeply and slowly

  o Humming and singing

  o Meditating

  o Eating omega-3 fatty acids (found in fish)

  o Consuming probiotics (try yogurt, traditional buttermilk, kefir, sauerkraut and other fermented foods)

  o Exercise

o   Try massage

These are all healthy things to work on regardless of your aim, but by stimulating the vagus nerve, you may be able to reap the benefits of reducing the amount of palpitations.

- ***Reduce your salt intake*** – Too much salt is not good for your health and may contribute to your palpitations. Make sure that you cut down on the amount of salt you consume throughout the day and be wary of added salt in packaged or processed foods. Eating a healthy diet overall can help reduce your menopausal symptoms and improve your health and general well-being.

- ***Drink plenty of water*** – Water is the magical elixir of life in so many ways. Make sure that you drink enough water every single day, without fail. There is some debate over how much is enough, but the general consensus is that eight glasses a day is sufficient. If you struggle with the bland taste, add a squeeze of fresh lemon and lime to jazz it up.

- ***Exercise regularly*** – Exercise is vital on so many levels. It helps to keep your heart healthy, regulates stress levels, reduces anxiety, and as a result, can help to reduce the number of palpitations you have, or even remove them completely. I suggest that you find a type of exercise that you enjoy and start doing it just a few hours per week. This is enough to keep you in better shape and the results will filter down through the rest of your body.

Natural Methods to Reduce Headaches:

- **Drink plenty of water** – Being dehydrated can cause a headache, so it might not even be your hormonal imbalance that is causing the pain, but the fact that you are dehydrated. Before reaching for a painkiller, sit down, relax and drink a glass of water. See how you feel after a short while. However, drinking plenty of water throughout the day, every day, will reduce the number of headaches you experience in general, whilst helping you to have more energy and even regulate your appetite.

- **Increase your magnesium intake** – You can take a magnesium supplement if you choose to, but you can go down the natural route and try getting your daily magnesium amount from your diet. Foods rich in magnesium include avocados, nuts, legumes, tofu, whole grains, seeds, and fatty fish types. You can also find magnesium in dark chocolate, but remember that moderation is vital as chocolate can also cause headaches in some people. If you feel like a supplement might be a better route for you, speak to your doctor before you begin, especially if you are currently taking any other medications or you have any pre-existing medical conditions. The green light from your doctor will give you peace of mind.

- *Cut down on alcohol intake* – Alcohol dehydrates your body, which is always going to lead to a headache. A hangover the next morning is partly down to dehydration, so remember to reduce your alcohol intake and see if your headaches decrease. This does not mean that you cannot enjoy the odd glass of wine, but it does mean that everything in moderation is the key. Alcohol is also a stimulant, so do not be tempted to drink an alcoholic drink before bed in the hope that it will help you sleep — it might help you nod off quicker but you will wake up during the night as the effects wear off, and you will probably need to get up and use the toilet more often, which is going to disrupt your sleep.

- *Make sure you get enough sleep* – Poor sleep is always going to lead to a headache and when you are not rested, a whole host of other problems come your way. Certainly, an insufficient amount of sleep and poor sleep quality are the main issues for menopausal women, but doing your best to try and get a regular seven to eight hours of sleep every night is important. Make sure that you go to bed and wake up at the same time every day, avoid stimulants (coffee, tea, smoking, alcohol) in the hours before bed, and lay off your phone usage an hour or so before you plan to sleep. Your sleeping environment needs to be comfortable ensuring that you are not too hot or too cold. Making an effort to improve your sleeping pattern is extremely important. Lack of sleep leads to sleep deprivation in the long-term and it must not be ignored. It does not just cause headaches, but can cause a myriad of other health issues too.

- *Avoid foods which have a high histamine amount* – Some women experience migraines or severe headaches when they eat a diet high in histamine. Histamine is a compound found within the body which cells release whenever you become ill or get injured. It is part of the immune system and encourages the inflammatory response. Histamine stimulates the dilation of capillaries within the body, which could lead to headaches. Cutting out foods high in histamine could therefore reduce your headaches naturally. Avoid fermented drinks, including alcohol (beer is the worst for this), fermented foods (including yogurt), avocados, dried varieties of fruit, eggplant, shellfish, smoked meat, processed meats, and spinach. You might look at that list and wonder why super-foods such as avocados and fermented foods, which are high in probiotics are there. It is because some women do not respond too well to these foods, therefore it is always a good idea to work out whether you fall into this bracket by cutting them out gradually one by one, and paying attention to how your body will respond to this change.

- *Use a cold compress* – Whilst you are suffering from a headache, try a cold compress across your head, with a glass of water on the side. Sit down with your head back and relax or lay down if you prefer. Close your eyes and focus on your breathing. You may find that after a short while the headache reduces without the need to take a painkiller. Make sure that the compress is not too cold, as this could cause the headache to worsen; cool is the aim here, not freezing.

- *Try essential oils* – Aromatherapy has been around for centuries, and the use of essential oils means that you can try and reduce many ailments without medical means; one of those ailments is headaches. Lavender oil, rosemary oil, peppermint oil, chamomile oil and eucalyptus oil are all recommended for reducing headaches and inflammation whilst lavender is also great for promoting sleep. You can add this to your bath water, place it on your wrists, spray a little onto your pillow, or simply inhale it via a diffuser.

- *B complex vitamins* – Some women find that taking a B complex vitamin supplement can help reduce the number of headaches they get, particularly migraines. If headaches are causing the issue for you, you can talk to your doctor about possibly adding this supplement to your routine. Alternatively, you can go down the natural route and add foods into your diet which are naturally high in this vitamin. These include salmon, liver, organ meats, eggs, leafy greens, milk, mussels, oysters, clams, beef, and legumes.

A few of the methods for reducing headaches are also useful for reducing the frequency of palpitations, and vice versa. However, the good news is that they are all quite easy to incorporate into your daily routine, and they will all give you other health benefits too.

Key Points

In this chapter, I have shared in-depth information about palpitations and headaches during the menopause. Again, not all women will find these symptoms to be a problem, but if they are troublesome for you, you can see that there are many natural ways to reduce them.

As with all the symptoms we have covered so far, headaches and palpitations during the menopause are mostly down to the hormonal fluctuations and imbalances you are experiencing during the perimenopause and the menopause phase. These can also continue after the menopause, for a few years into the postmenopausal period. If you are at all worried, you should go and see your doctor and get checked.

Whilst both of these symptoms are very common during the menopausal period, they are sometimes a sign of something a little more serious. Ruling that out will give you peace of mind, and from there you can work towards reducing these symptoms via natural means.

The main points to remember from this chapter are:

Headaches and palpitations are common symptoms during the menopause.

Not all women experience these symptoms, but many do. You could experience both symptoms together or separately, and one may be more severe than another.

- Palpations are rarely serious, but if you are worried, you should get them checked, as they could be a sign of a heart issue.

- Similarly, headaches are rarely severe, but they can be linked to other conditions, so if you are worried, get these checked with your doctor.

- Fluctuating hormone levels are the cause of both of these symptoms during this time of life.

- Stress can have a powerful effect on both palpitations and headaches, so naturally reducing stress is a good starting point.

- Both headaches and palpitations can be reduced via natural methods. Try to get enough sleep, drink plenty of water, and minimise exposure to stimulants.

Chapter 9

The Link With Osteoporosis

One of the main words that is associated with the menopause is "osteoporosis".

It may sound frightening, but when you dig a little deeper and understand more about it, you will realise that there are many things you can do to reduce your risk of developing osteoporosis in later life. It is also very unlikely that every menopausal woman is going to develop osteoporosis, but falling oestrogen levels do put you at a higher risk than at other times in your life. Women are also more at risk than men.

However, before we get into the finer details of how to minimise your risk, we need to delve a little deeper into what osteoporosis is.

What is Osteoporosis?

Osteoporosis is a long-term health problem that occurs as you age. Over time, bones weaken, and this makes them more likely to fracture and break more easily, than at any other time in life. The role of oestrogen helps to keep the bones strong and flexible, and the problem arises during the menopause when women start experiencing falling levels of oestrogen, which contributes to the risks of developing osteoporosis.

There is no routinely performed test to find out whether you are at risk of developing osteoporosis. It is usually diagnosed when someone breaks a bone, and a bone density test is done that shows whether or not you have osteoporosis. This is not routinely done beforehand, unless there is a medical indicator for it, in which case the doctor may send you for a DEXA scan. This measures the density of your bones and gives an indication of what is going on.

Osteoporosis affects all bones, but there are some more common ones — wrist, hips and vertebrae, also known as your spinal bones. We quite frequently hear about older people having hip replacements due to fractures and weakening. This can often be because of osteoporosis.

As with any medical condition, osteoporosis can be mild, moderate, or severe. In the worst cases, even a sneeze or a heavy cough can lead to a broken rib or having a problem with a spinal bone.

As osteoporosis sets in, your posture can change. You might have seen some elderly people in the forward bending position. This is due to osteoporosis, as the bones in the spine become weak and brittle, and therefore cannot support the body as well as they did before.

When osteoporosis is diagnosed, it can be treated with medicines that strengthen the bones, but the medication will not always work. This is why it is always best to look at prevention rather than attempting to cure what has been damaged. There is no actual cure for osteoporosis either, so a healthy lifestyle is one of the best ways to prevent this condition.

It sounds like a rather grim outlook, but it is important to mention that not every menopausal woman is going to develop osteoporosis when she gets older. This also is not a problem that is going to affect you right now; you will not know whether this is a problem for you until you notice regularly broken bones, a few years or even decades into the future.

How to Reduce Your Risk Factors for Osteoporosis

Whilst it is true that not every menopausal woman will develop osteoporosis in later life, it is something that you need to pay great attention to once you reach the postmenopausal stage. Osteoporosis can cause long-term pain when bones are weak and brittle, so you must do whatever you can right now to reduce this risk.

Both men and women can develop osteoporosis, but women are more likely to as a result of the loss of oestrogen during the menopause. This risk is further compounded if you undergo premature menopause or have had surgery to remove your ovaries.

So, what can you do to reduce the risk?

The good news is that there are steps you can start taking right now.

Regular Exercise

Regular exercise is the best starting point. Aim for around two and a half hours every week, hitting a moderate level of intensity. This can be walking fast, cycling, jogging, or anything that gets you out of breath and pushes your heart rate up.

You should also add in some weight bearing and resistance exercises, as these are ideal for boosting bone density, helping you reduce your risk of developing osteoporosis. Strength and flexibility are what you need to aim for.

I suggest you do some muscle strengthening exercises two to three days a week, and make sure that you use all the main muscle groups.

My book *Get Fit and Healthy in Your Own Home in 20 Minutes or Less*, which is available on Amazon, is a fantastic resource for finding exercise routines to suit your needs. Inside the book, you will find plenty of exercises that cover warm-ups, stretching, and strength training for your upper and lower body. You will also find many simple and healthy ideas for breakfast, lunch, dinner, and snacks.

The ideas for weight-bearing exercises include jogging, dancing, skipping, climbing stairs, and jumping up and down. Remember to wear shoes that give proper support to your feet and ankles. If you are having back problems or you struggle with your knees, then I recommend swimming as it is a less intense exercise, but it still gives your muscles a great workout.

On the other hand, resistance exercises look a little different. These include using hand weights, doing press-ups or lunges, etc. If you have gym membership, you will find plenty of equipment there to help you perform this type of exercise. Otherwise, you can usually make use of household items, for example two cans of food work very well for hand weights. There are many ideas for different types of exercises in my book, which I mentioned earlier.

Eat a Healthy Diet

So many of the menopausal symptoms we have looked at so far can be improved with eating healthily. A healthy diet is recommended as one of the main contributors to reducing the risks of osteoporosis.

Two main vitamins you need to help reduce your osteoporosis risk are calcium and vitamin D. Soon, I will talk about whether you can get these from a supplement, but first, let's explore natural methods.

Calcium helps to keep your bones healthy, as well as your teeth and nails. The recommended daily intake is 700mg per day and it is entirely possible to get that from your regular diet. Some of the foods which you can add to your daily diet include:

- Leafy greens (the darker, the better)

- Dried varieties of fruit

- Tofu

- Dairy products such as milk, cheese and yoghurt

Vitamin D works with calcium. It helps your body to absorb the calcium you are getting from food. Therefore, if you are deficient in vitamin D, the calcium you are consuming will not work efficiently.

Your daily intake of vitamin D needs to be 10 micrograms every day, and you can find vitamin D in the following foods:

- Red meat (it can increase your risk of heart disease when eaten in large quantities, therefore eat in moderation)

- Liver

- Oily varieties of fish such as herring, mackerel, sardines, and salmon

- Egg yolks

- Foods which are classified as "fortified", e.g. certain cereals — you will find this out by reading the packaging as it will be marketed as such

Increase Your Vitamin D Intake via Sunlight

It is possible to boost your own natural vitamin D production by soaking up the sun. Of course, you need to practice sun safety, as sunburn and sunstroke are not attractive or healthy. I recommend you go out and enjoy benefits of the sun when it is not as intense but is wonderfully warm.

Reduce Smoking and Drinking

Drinking alcohol and smoking can weaken bones over time and therefore contribute to your risk of developing osteoporosis. Smoking in particular has been shown to increase the likelihood of osteoporosis. As for drinking alcohol, it is recommended to stick to no more than 14 units per week to remain within healthy boundaries. Cutting down on drinking and stopping smoking can not only help you to prevent osteoporosis, but will also reduce many of your menopausal symptoms such as hot flushes.

Should You Take Supplements?

It is possible to take supplements for both calcium and vitamin D to support your bone health, but it is always a good idea to speak to your doctor about it, and understand the side effects of any supplement you are thinking of taking. As I mentioned earlier, calcium can generally be consumed in a sufficient amount for your body via your diet, but you may find it a little harder to get enough vitamin D following that route.

As suggested already, you can soak up the sun and increase your vitamin D production levels, but there are no concrete guidelines on how long it takes to be in the sun to give you enough of it. With that in mind, you might want to consider taking a vitamin D supplement alongside a healthy diet packed with a variety of different vitamins and minerals.

Key Points

In this chapter, you learnt how reduced oestrogen increases your risk of developing osteoporosis in later life. If you want to be happy and healthy in your later years, it is a good idea to start reducing your risk now.

Just because you are going through the menopause, it does not necessarily mean that you are going to develop osteoporosis, but it is a risk that you need to take seriously.

Here are the main points to remember from this chapter:

- Osteoporosis is the weakening of bones which typically happens in later life. It can occur as a result of low levels of oestrogen which contributes to your overall risk factor.

- Women who go through the menopause prematurely or who have had surgery to remove their ovaries have an increased risk.

- Osteoporosis varies in intensity and is indicated by the frequent breaking of bones, which can lead to long-term pain.

- Learning to reduce your risk of osteoporosis includes taking regular exercise, including moderate-level cardio, weight bearing and muscle strengthening exercises.

- Eating a healthy diet, packed with calcium and vitamin D, is important for strong and healthy bones.

- You can take a supplement of both vitamin D and calcium if you choose to.

- It is possible to boost your body's own vitamin D production by spending time in the sun.

Conclusion

Every woman goes through the menopause. It is not something you can shy away from or prevent, but you can control it in terms of whether it is a happy and healthy experience or a very difficult one. The menopause does not just happen to you. It is something you can shape to a certain degree and learn how to handle via natural ways, and in some cases, with a little help from the medical world.

You can make numerous lifestyle changes to help with standard and troubling menopausal symptoms, or you can choose to take the medication in the form of HRT. Never feel that you are being forced to take HRT as this is something you decide for yourself. Your doctor may encourage this as a good route for reducing the menopause symptoms, but if you are still unsure whether it is the best option for you, you do not have to take it.

There are many natural ways you can approach the issue and it is advisable to see how they work for you. Of course, you can always change your mind and ask for HRT again at a later stage if you are a suitable candidate for it.

The point is that you need to take control of your menopause and bend it to your will. It might sound impossible, but by reading this book you will hopefully have seen that it is entirely possible to do so. However, all of this requires a strong and positive mindset, with the determination to live a healthier and happier lifestyle.

A healthy and happy menopause is about focusing on your confidence and battling any troublesome symptoms. There is no "one size fits all" answer here, as every woman experiences a range of different symptoms, to varying degrees. What you can do, however, is read up on the most common and most troublesome symptoms and learn how to reduce their impact. The good news is that most of the advice for one troubling symptom will directly and positively impact many of the others. That means there is actually very little that you need to do, other than ensuring that your life in general is healthy and free of negative effects on your well-being.

Of course, that does not mean that you should just tolerate symptoms that are causing you problems. If you are struggling or you are worried about anything, you should speak to your doctor and seek reassurance and guidance. You may be going through the menopause for many years, and you might experience symptoms for up to 10 years — that is a lot of years to be dealing with symptoms that cause you discomfort or even distress. It is far better to speak to a health professional and find a way to reduce symptoms that trouble you, in a way that suits you. Thankfully, as you have learnt from this book, there are many options to choose from.

Every Woman's Experience is Different

I would like you to remember that every woman has a slightly different experience when going through the menopause. You can compare notes with your friends, but just because one friend is having a terrible time with mood swings, it does not mean that you will have a bad time too. Similarly, you might be troubled by hot flushes and night sweats, but she might barely notice them. You might be experiencing anxiety, but your sister may never have problems with it. There is no way to predict the symptoms you are going to have and which ones will be worse for you and which will be less troublesome.

We are all different and that is what makes us so wonderful. Unique women can take on the world and that also means taking on the menopause and conquering it, one symptom at a time.

However, it is a good idea to seek support from women going through the same thing as you and communicate with your loved ones and let them know what is going on. You are not in this alone, and the more you cut yourself off and try to handle it alone, the harder it will be. Share your experience to the degree you feel comfortable with and remember to be kind to yourself during this time. You are experiencing a lot of changes in your body and these are bound to affect how you feel within yourself and about yourself.

Your menopausal experience does not have to be negative, and it does not have to be a stage in your life that you just "get through". It can be a time to realise your power, to understand your body, and to reclaim what is yours. You no longer have to deal with those troublesome monthly bleeds, no more PMT, and you can wave goodbye to pregnancy risk! Once the menopause is over, none of these things are a concern anymore and whilst you might still have symptoms for a few years afterwards, you can rest safe in the knowledge that they will not last forever. Whether that is a few months more or a few years more depends entirely on your body, but they will disappear in the end.

Hopefully you will have absorbed all the information in this book and understood what you need to do to make your menopausal journey easier.

I also hope that you learnt enough about health and well-being to pass that information onto your family members. Just because they are not going through the menopause, it does not mean they should not focus on health! When the entire household is eating healthily, it is far easier for you to do it too and stick to it. You will notice that with the support of your family, you will be able to get through your menopausal journey much more easily.

Final Words

I want to say that we must not simply blame hormones for everything that happens to us. It is very easy to say "I'm fat because of my hormones", or "I'm stressed because of my hormones", or "I'm tired because of my hormones".

Yes, your hormones can affect your weight, mood and sleep, but paying attention to your diet, lifestyle and changing your attitude and behaviour towards the way you live your life, will significantly impact your hormones and your general well-being. Do not allow your hormones to control you. Make sure that you control YOU.

All that is left to do now is to wish you a healthy and happy menopause, full of empowerment, confidence, and the realisation that you are a truly unique and special woman who is not defined by the time of life she is going through.

Keep this book handy and refer to it whenever a new symptom comes your way, or whenever you want to change your approach to an existing one. Consider it your guide to achieving a happy, healthy, and perhaps even confidence-boosting menopause!

I wish you all the best!

Lots of love xx

Silvana

Thank You

I hope you enjoyed this book!

Please consider leaving a review on Amazon. Even if it is only a few sentences, it would be a huge help.

Here is the link for your convenience. Go to http://viewbook.at/manage-menopause. Your review will help other readers benefit from the information in this book.

Please visit bit.ly/silvana-signup to join the mailing list for updates on future books and to receive information about health, weight loss, and nutrition.

About the Author

Silvana Siskov has spent more than 20 years working with people experiencing a variety of issues, such as mental health, eating disorders and weight management problems. Her speciality is giving sound advice with a strong focus on emotional support. She is also dedicated to helping clients find a strong direction in the areas of their lives where they need it the most.

Silvana helps establish clarity around the issues which her clients are facing in their everyday lives. This allows them to take control of their health and well-being and change their lifestyle towards the positive end of the scale. By doing this, they are able to achieve their own health goals and improve their confidence levels and develop a sense of self-worth.

Following some personal health issues, Silvana's interest in nutrition grew. This led her towards supporting clients on their weight loss journeys, giving them advice on nutrition and their dietary needs and helping them overcome pitfalls such as comfort eating.

From this experience, Get Your Sparkle Back: 10 Steps to Weight Loss and Overcoming Emotional Eating was born. The fantastic reaction to this book led her to write more, helping her clients to achieve their own lifestyle goals and feel more confident from within. The book *Live Healthy on a Tight Schedule* followed quickly, empowering readers to be far less dependent on external factors and to take more control of their lives. Shortly after this book was published, *Get Fit and Healthy in Your Own Home in 20 Minutes or Less* was written. This book continues to help Silvana's readers to work towards their health and weight loss goals.

The following two books that Silvana wrote were focused on the menopause. The first book in the series *Beat Your Menopause Weight Gain*, was very quickly followed by *Free Yourself From Hot Flushes and Night Sweats*. With these two books Silvana helps women to better manage their menopausal journey and to reduce symptoms brought by the menopause.

Silvana finds true pleasure in supporting her clients and working closely with them on a one-on-one basis. She also extends her work into the community, with talks and workshops for those who prefer a more sociable atmosphere.

Silvana's overall mission is to empower and motivate women, helping them to use their power from within and create a deeper connection to themselves. By doing so, they can achieve whatever they put their minds to, living their very best lives.

Helpful Resources

Books by Silvana Siskov:

- *"Get Your Sparkle Back: 10 Steps to Weight Loss and Overcoming Emotional Eating."* The book is available on Amazon. Go to http://viewbook.at/sparkle.

- *"Live Healthy on a Tight Schedule: 5 Easy Ways for Busy People to Develop Sustainable Habits Around Food, Exercise and Self-Care."* The book is available on Amazon. Go to http://viewbook.at/livehealthy.

- *"Get Fit and Healthy in Your Own Home in 20 Minutes or Less: An Essential Daily Exercise Plan and Simple Meal Ideas to Lose Weight and Get the Body You Want."* The book is available on Amazon. Go to http://viewbook.at/get-fit.

- *"Get Fit and Healthy on a Tight Schedule 2 Books in 1."* The book is available on Amazon. Go to http://viewbook.at/get-fit2books.

- *"Break the Binge Eating Cycle: Stop Self-Sabotage and Improve Your Relationship With Food."* The book is available on Amazon. Go to http://viewbook.at/breakthebinge.

- *"Relaxation and Stress Management Made Simple: 7 Proven Strategies to Calm Your Mind, Stop Negative Thinking and Improve Your Life."* The book is available on Amazon. Go to http://viewbook.at/stressfree.

Free Mini-Courses:

- *Discover 10 Secrets of Successful Weight Loss*

- *This is How to Start Eating Less Sugar*

- *Learn How to Boost Your Energy – 11 Easy Ways*

- *Your Guide to a Happy and Healthy Menopause*

- *This is How to Lose Weight in Your 40's and Beyond*

Free Courses Available at:

www.silvanahealthandnutrition.com/course/